Maybe Baby

Navigating The Emotional Journey Through Assisted Fertility

Sue Saunders

16pt

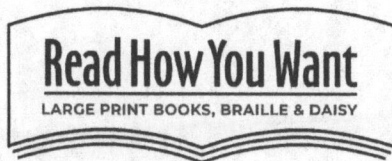

Read How You Want

LARGE PRINT BOOKS, BRAILLE & DAISY

Copyright Page from the Original Book

TABLE OF CONTENTS

For all those on the journey towards having a child.

I hope this book provides support and comfort.

DISCLAIMER

This book includes the author's personal account of dealing with infertility and grief. It also includes other stories that do not belong to any one individual or couple but represent the common issues that arise during counselling.

This book does not replace counselling. It is intended to help inform and support people and to be used alongside professional services.

Acknowledgements

Writing this book has been a pleasure, not least of all as I have had occasion to recall the many remarkable people I have encountered in my time as a fertility counsellor. These people include the clients who shaped my working career, my fellow fertility counsellors whose caring and support for me and each other was unfailing and consistent, the staff of the various clinics who supported me and gently took me in hand when I was getting a bit obsessive about one or other issue, Fertility Associates who provided me with many opportunities to develop as a counsellor and person, and my friends who have showed interest in and support for this book. My thanks to you all.

There are many people who have contributed to this book in a variety of ways. My biggest thanks go to my husband Alan and our daughters, without them I would be a lesser person. They have generously supported me throughout while accepting that my experience is also their experience. Being infertile was life-changing for me but not quite as life-changing as becoming a parent six years after the first diagnosis. Alan has stood by me through the turbulence of infertility, and has been a great partner and dad as our daughters have grown up and become adults. His support and encouragement have made writing this second book a pleasure. Thank you, Alan, for being my partner in life and for our good lives together. With Alan and the girls' consent I have shared our story in the Introduction.

I had the remarkably good fortune to work for Fertility Associates for nearly 20 years. At Fertility Associates Hamilton I was superbly managed by Batami Pundak, who cared for me in a professional, kind and loyal manner, and I was lucky to work with professional, competent, supportive and fun staff. It was a pleasure to work for this firm, whose values and ethics are strong with the care of patients foremost in their minds. Joi Ellis guided me through my own fertility journey and along with Margaret Stanley Hunt has been a confidante, colleague and friend. Margaret and Dr Mary Birdsall agreed to review this book and advise me along the way. I am very thankful to these two wonderful women for this support and interest.

Without clients there would be no fertility clinics. It has been my privilege to meet and work with many fine and courageous people. I always hoped that at the end of every counselling session the client(s) would feel thoroughly listened to and may have acquired some ideas or knowledge that might help them move forward. I like people and have felt lucky to work in such a trusting way with them.

Penguin Random House published my first book in 1998. When I approached them to pass the rights to that book back to me, Margaret Sinclair asked what I hoped to do with it. This proved to be a seminal question. I thank Margaret and her colleagues at Penguin Random House for providing just the right level of support through the writing stage and beyond.

I wish you, the reader, well, and hope your dreams are able to be fulfilled.

Sue Saunders

Introduction

In the 1980s, my husband Alan and I decided we would like to have children. We recognised it could take a while but decided that if it happened quickly we would be able to cope. So we stopped contraception and we began hoping. We had friends who had been down the route of unsuccessfully trying to have a child and had witnessed their sadness and pain, and hoped this was not our lot also. After a year of trying we headed to the GP and had some initial tests, and all seemed to be okay until it was found that my fallopian tubes were blocked. With the problem identified we were referred to Auckland for microsurgery, which was the only option as in vitro fertilisation (IVF) was not readily available in New Zealand at the time. We hoped after the surgery all would be well, and indeed I seemed to conceive readily. But sadly I miscarried many pregnancies and Alan and I began to adjust to our lives without children. We were both moving forward in our careers and decided to focus on that for a while. I did some further counselling training and set up a private practice.

My sense of myself as a woman was challenged, and fortunately Alan was reassuring. Yet the shadow of my infertility and grief stayed with me and my envy of those parenting was always present. I was open with people about our infertility and talked with some groups about the grief of infertility and the strategies we were using to cope. Through one of these talks, we were offered a child to adopt, who became our elder daughter. Her birth mother, also a Sue, was 36 weeks pregnant. She gave us the greatest gift of becoming parents after six years of trying. We remain firmly connected with her, and our daughter has always known of Sue's place in her and our lives.

A few months after we adopted we became pregnant and this time I held the pregnancy for 30 weeks. Our second daughter was born weighing under a kilogram and having to fight to stay alive. Our two daughters have been our joy since.

*

WHEN WE DISCOVERED I had fertility problems I sought information through reading. I learn, and am comforted, by reading and talking, as are many people. Those were the days before the internet, and I quickly discovered that there was almost nothing available. Finally I came across Barbara Eck Menning's 1977 book, which I had sent over from the USA. I carried this book with me to refer to it when I felt unsure, and it reassured me for the six years until we became parents.

My role as a counsellor, first in education and then in private practice, stood me in good stead and I seemed to attract clients with fertility issues. My own first book, *Infertility: A Guide for New Zealanders,* was written in the days when there was little available about infertility in New Zealand. Not long after publication a job became available in a leading fertility clinic in New Zealand and I applied. At this time I had been a counsellor for nearly two decades and had written in the fertility field. I accepted the role of fertility counsellor in early 2001. During my 20 years in the role, I was aware that less than a quarter of the clients who attended the clinic made use of the counselling service. One woman commented that she would rather read at home about how infertility would affect them. But there was not a lot written about the emotional impact and how to cope with infertility, so she came to counselling to find out if she was the only one with these feelings and how she could get through this experience and still function well within her life. At the end she said, 'Why don't you write this down for everyone? We all need the opportunity to access information in the way that suits us.'

And so this second book came about. My hope is that when someone picks up the book they will dip into the sections that are relevant or of interest to them rather than trying to read the whole book. Some people might find they start in one place, put the book down and as treatment develops read a different section. I hope the families and friends of the people struggling to be parents might find this book useful also.

*

EVERYONE HAS HARD experiences in their lives; infertility is simply one of the hardest of all. The wish to parent is a biological drive as well as an emotional desire. When someone who is experiencing infertility sees the joy created by others' news about a pregnancy or the birth of a baby, they wonder if they will ever feel this joy. What is a joy for others brings sadness and despair for those wanting to be parents, who may feel excluded from the experience and from belonging to a group of people called parents, whom our society values.

As they should, pregnant people and new parents become thoroughly engaged by the miracle that is happening for them. For new mothers, especially, the child becomes their life as they care for him or her, and it is the topic of conversation they enjoy most of all. It becomes difficult for the new parents to maintain the earlier levels of variety of conversation and activity with their non-parenting friends. Their lives now focus around being a parent and their baby's needs.

At work, we constantly see both female and male workers taking parental leave and sharing photos and news of their children, and with workplaces largely open-plan these days, it is hard to avoid hearing these conversations. Holidays such as Easter and Christmas are often child-dominated, and many work functions involve employees' children, which can be extremely hard for those of us who have, so far, had no luck becoming parents.

All people experiencing fertility problems are different; each person will have needs and ways of being that are particular and personal to them. Some couples wish to find others with similar fertility issues, hoping to develop new friendships within the infertile community. One out of four couples have some level of fertility challenge, so it is relatively easy to make connections, and the consumer group Fertility New Zealand has support groups in most main towns in New Zealand.

Many couples begin by sharing their situation with a few confidants within their family or friends and getting the support they need there. This may be an entirely new situation to all the people they talk with, but the support they reach out for will help them manage their lives. Other couples are private and wish to deal with infertility largely on their own. There is no right or wrong about these coping styles. Each style has benefits and disadvantages—probably the most important aspect is that the couple talk to each other and agree on how they will approach the issue.

There will be some people who wish to have lots of information about what is happening to them and the treatments they are offered. They feel knowledge will improve their capacity to do the treatment successfully and to understand what the medical staff are talking about. Others feel knowing too much and understanding the risks and successes of treatment will raise their anxiety and they instead wish to proceed knowing just the basics and trusting staff.

Undertaking fertility treatment will create a raft of emotions for every person, including uncertainty, confusion, anxiety, sadness, fear, hope and quite often joy. Staying strong and caring for yourself and each other is important. There are suggestions of things to think about and things people can do to take care of themselves both within and at the end of chapters.

My hope is that I have been able to recognise and include the many different groups who use fertility services. In the time I have worked as a fertility counsellor, single women making the decision to parent by themselves rather than miss out, and same-gender female couples, have become frequent users of the clinics, and in recent years there has been an increase in the number of same-gender male couples. These people seek the help of a donor and, in the case of men, a surrogate. They come to the clinic like any other couple, needing the skills and help of the clinic to become parents. Their journey is often more complex than that of heterosexual couples. There are sections within this book that provide information specific to each of these situations. Each clinic also helps a range of different ethnicities and cultures, and I hope I have acknowledged some of the issues faced by various cultures within this book.

I hope that as you read this book you find information, ideas and suggestions throughout that will help you maintain your sense of self and connection to the world. The book is not a replacement for counselling, it is an addition to the expert help the counsellors provide. I hope the book works alongside your treatment to support you, and provides comfort and help as you proceed through your journey.

Infertility changes the way people see the world. It challenges assumptions about having children and being parents. And it challenges and may change your relationships with family and your friends. It seldom only affects the people in the midst of the experience. As with anything we do in the world, if this is your pathway, make it work for you. Become informed and make the lifestyle changes that will support you along the journey and enhance your chances of becoming a parent. I wish you well in the journey and hope the outcome will provide you with a life you can embrace.

Chapter 1

Learning about infertility

Most people assume they can have a family when they wish. The dawning realisation that it may be difficult creates a sense of distance between their expectations and reality. This distance extends to their relationships with significant family and friends, who may have conceived easily. People seldom have any prior knowledge of problems, so they need information and expertise in order to resolve the issue themselves.

Jenny and Bryn

JENNY: Two years ago we had the best life we could imagine. We had planned things and everything had gone just right. We loved each other, and still do, so much. Life was good then. Bryn and I belong to a group of friends who have known each other for years and see lots of each other on weekends. We were one of the last of the group to marry and buy a home, and we delayed trying for children until we felt secure.

BRYN: Yes, we wanted everything right before we dropped to one income, and I wanted Jenny to have the opportunity to stay home longer than just the maternity leave if she wished. She is so good with our friends' children and we knew this was to be a very happy phase of our lives together.

JENNY (through tears): We were always out of sync with our friends and I lived through the women all talking about their first pregnancies and births, but I managed that because our turn was coming up. Now we are a whole child behind, and with them expecting number two I can't manage to sit through all that again and not join in. They don't talk about anything else. So I feel as if I am losing my friends as well as our dream.

BRYN (keeping a tight arm around her shoulder to comfort her): I really don't know how to make this better for Jenny. The men don't talk about the pregnancies and children much at all so I don't get that, but every time we go out Jenny weeps all the way home and now does not want to go to barbeques or outings with the group.

JENNY: We have been trying for 18 months and have just seen the doctor here at the clinic today. We both have issues but our results don't give enough answers so we have to do more tests. She says we score for public funding but the wait is one and a half to two years. I can't wait that long. I am already nearly 35 and Bryn is 37. We want more than one child and don't want to be old parents.

I feel so sad and so angry—I work with children and I see parents who do not seem to appreciate their children, and here we are, desperate to have children. Where is the justice in that? I hate feeling like this and just want to feel happy again. It's been a long time since I just felt happy.

Finding someone to love and share our life with is one of life's hopes for most of us. We look for a person who fits our needs and who we can enjoy life with. The time of developing and consolidating a relationship is generally positive. In this time we get to know each other, find out about each other's ways of living, discuss goals and dreams and develop mutual pathways for the future. For a high proportion of couples, having a family is one of the goals they share.

When the time comes to try for a pregnancy most people are aware that when they stop contraception it may take them a while to conceive. They don't worry too much for the first six months but enjoy the intimacy of making love and the hope it will begin a baby. Each period is a time of disappointment, followed by the hope of the next cycle. By six months they start to think they should be getting pregnant and may do some research and discover the Fertility New Zealand or a similar group's statement: 'A couple is regarded as having a fertility problem when they have not conceived after 12 months of regular unprotected sexual intercourse.'

Understanding this statement is a starting point for looking into what may be happening for them. Within New Zealand there is sound information provided both by Fertility New Zealand, the consumer support group, and the fertility clinics, which have accessible and informative websites. Reading may help the couple understand when it is appropriate to seek help or, if in early days, to ensure they are maximising their opportunities, such as making love around the time of ovulation. For some people, looking into some of the alternative treatments is their beginning point.

Couples where the woman is over 35 should consider talking to a fertility specialist after six months of trying unsuccessfully. Couples where the woman is under 35 may approach a clinic after a year. Timing can be important for ensuring good-quality eggs.

Infertility affects one out of four heterosexual couples in New Zealand. While some people are prepared to keep trying for longer by themselves, about two-thirds will approach a clinic to see the specialist and look for a solution. Of these couples about 40 per cent have a female issue—low egg reserve, ovulation issues, endometriosis or polycystic ovaries are the common problems. Another 40 per cent have male issues, such as low sperm count or unusual morphology (sperm shape).

Being part of the remaining 20 per cent is perhaps the most frustrating. In this case it may be a combined factor with issues for both the man and the woman, or the doctors may not be able to find a reason for the lack of pregnancy.

Then there is social infertility, which is experienced by gay couples, transgender people and single people. The desire to parent and the grief at having to involve others in baby-making is just as great for these people, and their need for support and treatment is similar to heterosexual couples. Other groups of people who need or choose to use clinics to have a child include couples with a known genetic issue they would like to avoid passing onto their children (see 'Genetic conditions'), and couples with one or more existing children who are not achieving a subsequent pregnancy (see 'Chapter 16: Secondary infertility').

Regardless of the reason, infertility hurts and impacts on each person's life in different ways. Having to admit to needing help, and then exposing their intimate lives to doctors, nurses, embryologists and counsellors, is painful.

My own experience as an infertile woman is similar to the experience of most infertile women and men. I didn't want it, didn't enjoy it, and only in retrospect can I say I benefited. I believe infertility is unwelcome for any couple. It affects their self-esteem, it intrudes into and dominates their lives, it takes away their privacy and affects their friendships and extended families.

Infertility and heterosexual couples

Most people grow up with the assumption they will be able to be parents in a timely manner. Fortunately a high portion of people are able to achieve this. The people who are unable to achieve this have impacts that often last for the rest of their lives. Women may have constructed a career that allows for parental leave and part-time work so they can manage their family as it grows. Men may have visualised themselves guiding their children through life or coaching their child's soccer team. Both are likely to have dreams and visions that feel important to them, which they have shared with their partner. From the time they begin to realise they will not achieve a pregnancy easily these dreams and hopes become precarious.

Learning to talk to each other and others about these fears and losses is often a new experience for couples. It involves sharing at a level that feels private—our internal thoughts and feelings, our dreams and fears. Largely we hold these inside ourselves, and to expose them, even to our partner, is to expose a core of our self and to feel vulnerable. For a portion of people even discussing the menstrual cycle and ovulation will be new conversations, especially for some men. Being gentle with each other and not allowing hurt to override communication while having these discussions can help both people to talk about how it is for them. While it is important to understand how the reproductive systems work, equally it is important for both people to talk about the feelings they are coping with.

One of the first casualties for a couple may be their lovemaking. Most heterosexual couples begin with lovemaking as an expression of their attraction for each other and their pleasure in being together as a couple. As they try for children the purpose changes, and this affects the frequency and timing of the lovemaking. In an effort to start a pregnancy, intercourse is more frequent around the ovulation time of the month and this may mean it is less frequent in other times. The reason for making love has changed and so too has the sexual pleasure in each other. It may not, at the beginning, diminish the frequency in making love, but as time increases and a couple is unsuccessful in becoming pregnant their concept of just enjoying making love may vanish.

Most of us are brought up to believe that if we want something enough we should try hard to get it, practise a lot, and if we don't succeed try a bit harder. When applied to infertility, this can be very frustrating and disheartening. Most couples trying for a pregnancy and not having success begin to time their lovemaking and forget about enjoying sex for the rest of the month. Both men and women become aware of the predicted ovulation time in some way—a calendar, using the ovulation prediction app on their phone or through the use of ovulation kits. This timing of sex has the potential to become obsessive, and instead of making love they have a 'job' to be done each month. Couples may talk about the timing to make love but seldom mention the impact it is having on their feelings about sex. Their pleasure and performance often suffers, with satisfaction or orgasm harder to achieve. Most couples, when asked gently about this in counselling, will acknowledge the impact of their infertility on their pleasure in and frequency of sex. Most are relieved it is out in the open and want to talk about how to manage this.

Counselling sessions where sexual issues are discussed can provide a significant change for couples. Sort of an 'aha' moment. By both the man and the woman expressing their feelings of frustration, inadequacy and their fear that pregnancy may not happen, they give themselves and their partner insight into the impact this is having on each of them and as a couple. The value of a facilitated discussion with the counsellor supporting and helping them be clear and honest allows a greater understanding of each other.

It is sometimes useful for the couple to reflect on the beginning of their relationship, recollecting times when they enjoyed themselves as a couple in areas such as their social lives as well as their intimate lives. It is useful for them to think about what it was that drew them together at the beginning and the activities they enjoyed while dating. By reminding themselves of their earlier, generally happy, pre-baby-making days they may consider bringing forward some of the feelings, activities and intimacy that allowed them to enjoy their times together without the focus being their lack of pregnancy.

There are a variety of feelings that people can struggle with at the beginning of their effort to become pregnant. A sense of guilt is often felt by both parties even before they know the reason for their struggle. Self-blame makes it hard for a woman or man to function well within a relationship, and the sense of optimism and initiation of activities suffers when a person is consumed by guilt. There may be a feeling of shame involved. Shame is a powerful emotion, and is often hidden. A person might fear that something that has happened in the past, such as a sexually transmitted disease or termination of pregnancy, is the cause for their lack of success in babymaking, and this can cause feelings of shame. Sometimes the fear they might lose their partner if they share is strong, other times they may not have the language to express themselves well. It takes a lot of courage to admit to guilt or shame and ask for help to resolve it. Having support and someone to help both parties communicate about these feelings may be helpful. Sometimes friends or family may be confidants, other times this may feel too personal to share with people who are so close.

It is hard for both parties to discuss the worry that they may not be able to provide a baby for the relationship. Both societal and cultural expectations may lead to the belief that a marriage has greater worth when there is a child. Many see fertility as the responsibility of women. Fortunately an increasing number of men recognise the injustice in placing this responsibility onto the woman. As mentioned earlier, fertility problems occur roughly equally in men and in women, and in some relationships the reason may belong to both, or be unable to be identified.

There are generally gender differences in the desire to sort out why pregnancy is not happening. Women often feel a greater urgency about becoming a parent and may be the driver to change lovemaking to around their ovulation time. They are also likely to be the person who initiates seeking help from their GP or a fertility clinic. This seems to relate to their knowledge that fertility is affected by increasing age, especially for women. Men support their partner in the plan to have children but may become confused about how quickly it escalates to becoming a problem that they need help to sort out. They may feel resentment about the impact it has had on their sex lives but not feel able to speak about this to their partners.

One of the challenging things for men is seeing the stress their partners feel as a result of not achieving pregnancy and feeling powerless to help change this. Societal stereotypes say that men should stay strong and support their partner. This may mean the man hides his own emotions and does not talk about the problem. He does this not because he is not feeling frustrated and sad about the situation, but because he feels this will support the woman he loves. But being staunch may in fact not be helpful to the woman, who most likely just wants to know that her partner shares her sadness and despair at the situation. Some men have been brought up without a good language for feelings and may be uncomfortable having discussions about how they feel. Women, who often have been brought up to talk about emotions and problems, wish they could have a long conversation with their partner about how they can cope together and what helps each person. It is important to recognise that these conversations are difficult to have, and attempting to talk about it constantly may not be helpful. If the talks are unsatisfactory, both people will dread trying again. It is useful for couples to limit the time and frequency of these talks and to ensure life still has good times as well as problem-solving.

Communication is different for men and women. As a generalisation, women tend to talk about their feelings more, repeating the same thing, and in hearing themselves saying things they refine their language and process information, enabling them to move forward. This can be frustrating for men, who may process information internally and need time to consider what they have heard. This mismatch may cause tension within the couple.

A woman may have confided in a family member or friend to talk about the problem the couple are experiencing. She may do this prior to talking to her partner, and as a result she is more experienced in understanding and expressing her feelings. Men will often mull the issues over during their day but not share their feelings. This imbalance in readiness to talk, especially about feelings, can lead to communication difficulties and reluctance to communicate. One way of trying to get more balance and readiness in the conversation is to decide, for example, 'This evening we will spend half an hour talking about how we feel about not getting pregnant.' This decision can be made prior to talking to give each person time to think about what they want to talk about. Any discussion should be with the TV, computer and phones off so the couple can concentrate on each other. This is a personal, in-depth conversation in which both the man and the woman will feel vulnerable at times and need the support of their partner.

As a suggestion, it is often easier to have these conversations when walking or driving. This way the couple are alongside each other and not in opposition, facing each other, as they usually are when sitting in chairs. Movement also may help the couple to progress the discussion rather than getting stuck.

Many couples find the changes in their relationship and communication disconcerting and hard to deal with. They began their lives together having fun, talking and planning for the future. As time goes on and they find they are not achieving a pregnancy they may find they are not equipped to cope with troubles and differences in opinion. Listening and accepting there may be differences is showing respect to your partner. Learning to listen well requires that we harness our own feelings and allow the other person to talk about how it is for them. Just allowing them to talk without interruptions tells them that we care about how they are feeling. Indeed we can't tell others how to feel, we can only tell them how we feel and then listen to how they feel. By being allowed to say how it is for them and to hear an alternative, people will often move forward when the topic is next discussed.

Social infertility

Social infertility is the term used when referring to infertility caused by a lack of either eggs or sperm for a single person, for a gay couple, or for trans people who wish to parent. Socially infertile people may not be medically infertile, but they cannot start a pregnancy by circumstance or relationship—they need gametes (eggs and sperm) from another person to create a baby. Donor sperm is needed for same-gender female couples and single women, and donor eggs plus surrogacy is required for same-gender male couples and single men. The desire to parent can be strong for these people, and the pathway to parenting may be long and complicated.

Many gay, trans and single people have the same desires as other people to nurture children, to have children in their daily lives and to form a family that includes children to parent. Fortunately New Zealand society as a whole is becoming less discriminatory and the clinics are inclusive in providing treatment to these people. There are some differences in access as most socially infertile people will not score enough medical points to entitle them to public funding.

While there are feelings of frustration and sadness at having to take the path through a clinic to become a parent, the majority are also relieved they have access to medically and legally safe processes. The longing to be a parent can be the beginning of a long journey through finding a donor (see Chapter 12), and for men also finding a surrogate (see Chapter 15), then accessing the treatment. For single women and single men the added grief of not having a partner to share the parenting may complicate their feelings around needing a donor.

Some couples decide to seek a donor or a surrogate through the internet and to create a child without the use of the clinics. This process has a level of risk, and the hopeful parents place a lot of trust in the donating person and/or the surrogate. Usually sperm donors who meet people on the web are strangers, and as a result of communication and home inseminations they have access to the families they have helped create. While many are kind and trustworthy people there have been instances in New Zealand of donors who have harassed the new family and wanted access to the women or children in ways that far exceeded the initial agreement. In a number of cases this has led to expensive court cases to get a level of safety for the family, so caution should be taken.

Amanda

Amanda wanted to try for a child while she still had some chance of succeeding. She enquired about the use of donor sperm through the clinic and got onto the waiting list, but at the time it was nearly two years. She then decided to explore finding a man who might donate to her privately using 'turkey basting', or home insemination.

She went onto a website she understood had some donors and began her search there. She was unsure about this process so began talking with others in her online group about home insemination with an unknown donor. The information she received was frightening—a couple of regular donors were not respecting the women or their families.

Amanda withdrew from the online donor site and went about finding a personal donor to reduce the waiting time. She asked a number of trusted girlfriends if they could help her, and one had a male friend she trusted who was willing to be a donor providing he was not a liable parent to the child.

The potential donor requested they do the donation through the clinic to protect all parties. Amanda agreed and the process took about six months before she could have her treatment, which was successful.

Where surrogacy for a same-gender male couple happens outside of the clinic, with a surrogate using her eggs, which are inseminated by a man's sperm, there is a large amount of trust. Trust from the woman that the man or men will support her in the pregnancy, that they will take the baby at birth and later adopt the child to become the legal parents, and that they will be good parents. It is also about trust from the men that the woman will not make unusual financial demands and will relinquish the child for them to adopt. Currently, the men have no legal rights until they adopt the baby, so they will need to be sure of the surrogate. Some people use a woman they know or who is connected to them through friends—although not foolproof, this helps protect all parties and safeguards the child. Trust and safety for all parties and especially the children are important.

Increasingly same-gender couples, single and trans people are using the clinic to create a child and feeling positive about the safety and the legality this places around them. The required counselling for these treatments provides them with a good basis for understanding the process and the emotional aspects of treatment. They also receive ongoing support throughout the experience.

Genetic conditions

Some people come to the clinic because of a known genetic condition that they wish to avoid passing on to children. There is a pathway that will help these people work through this, and by using genetic testing, such as preimplantation genetic diagnosis (PGD), they can avoid passing their condition onto their child.

PGD is used for serious genetic disorders, such as cystic fibrosis. Very often people find these genetic disorders when they have an initial child who is affected, and they wish to avoid this in subsequent children. Sometimes they will be aware, through their family history, that there is a disorder to avoid.

The process begins with a discussion with the fertility doctor. The doctor will talk about PGD's relevance to the person's case and the processes that are necessary, including costs. The process will also involve a genetic counsellor, the clinic counsellor and a feasibility study to identify the genes involved. Often this treatment has government funding associated with it.

PGD begins with IVF. Instead of having an embryo replaced at day five, a biopsy or removal of a few cells from each embryo is performed and the cells sent away for testing. The embryos are frozen and the couple awaits their results. They are allowed to use embryos that are unaffected or carriers of the condition. The Ministry of Health, which funds treatment, do not allow the use of affected embryos.

IVF with PGD is a long process, and the couple will have periods of inaction and waiting, which can prove stressful and raise anxiety. One of the reasons the clinic counsellor is involved is to help couples plan for this and for unexpected results.

The second way of testing the genetic viability of embryos is preimplantation genetic screening (PGS). This technique may be used by people to check that the correct number of chromo somes are present in their embryos. It is often suggested to people over 35. Sometimes PGS is used by people with a large number of embryos to help in embryo selection. If there have been repeated implantation failures or miscarriages, PGS may be used to check the viability of the embryos.

As with PGD, those who wish to use PGS will need to do IVF and have cells biopsied from their embryos for testing. The embryos will be frozen until the results tell which embryos are the best to use.

There are some situations in which testing is not allowed by New Zealand law. The most often questioned one is for sex selection, which is illegal.

Things to think about

- What impact has not getting pregnant had on you, or, if in a relationship, on each of you as well as on your relationship?
- How well are you able to communicate about these tricky issues?
- Who else is okay to confide in if you need to?
- What resources have you located? Do you need more?
- Are you using resources that are relevant to the New Zealand situation?
- What do you know about donations and surrogacy if you need them?
- Should you look on a website, either FertilityNZ or one of the clinics', to gain more information?

Things that might be helpful

- Maintaining a level of exercise to help alleviate stress and to feel healthy.
- Finding out about lifestyle factors that influence fertility and activating them.
- Being very gentle with each other and allowing your partner to have a bad day and for you to support them.
- Reading specifically about the issues you may need to talk with the doctor about.
- Joining FertilityNZ and finding out what they have to offer—information, support.
- Distracting yourself with things that have nothing to do with fertility to stop it from taking over your lives: watching movies or series on TV, sport, gardening, DIY—anything that is outside of yourself.

Chapter 2

Grief—the ongoing story

All clients who experience infertility will experience a grief reaction: with infertility comes loss, and with loss comes grief. (Deveraux and Hammerman, *Infertility and Identity: New Strategies for Treatment.*)

Many of us are very child-focused; we see parenthood as a rite of passage into true adulthood. We may see parenting as an opportunity to relive our childhood. We know society, our families and cultures expect us to have children and value the children as an extension of ourselves. We assume that we will be able to fulfil these desires.

Trying for a child is an exciting time in a couple's life. But as the months go by and periods still arrive, anxiety creeps in. A bit more time of trying and fear comes along—fear that something is wrong and a pregnancy won't occur.

Some people at this point begin to research, maybe on the web, about things they can do to help themselves. Life begins to rotate around monthly cycles of ovulation times and awaiting a period. Each period brings a sense of loss, another month lost, the dreams about the creation of their child fades, and with it comes a concern that they may need help.

Some keep trying for extended periods of time as the sense of disbelief that anything could be wrong counters the concern that is just below the surface. The hope that begins every month can provide a balance to the sadness felt with the arrival of a period. Sometimes this sadness is discounted or seen as hormonal. It is more useful to recognise sadness as a loss of the hope and dream for that month.

Laura and Mike

Laura found the lead-up to her periods almost unmanageable. She became anxious, tearful and some months felt unable to work effectively. Once her period arrived she settled down again. She had decided it was premenstrual tension, but since she was trying to get pregnant she did not want to take anything for it.

Mike became very concerned about her, and felt unable to help her manage. He suggested they go to their doctor together. This turned out to be the right decision as the GP listened carefully and suggested they seek specialist advice, both about the reason they were not conceiving and about managing the anxiety this was causing.

Within the couple each person may have different feelings. Women, with their menstrual cycles, have hormonal swings within each month. They tend to know when ovulation then periods occur, and consequently are very aware of their lack of pregnancy. When the decision is made to have a child, the woman often begins to see the changes this will bring to her life and work and to anticipate these with pleasure. So the arrival of her period signals not only that she is not pregnant for the month but also that her life and work changes are not about to happen.

Gender differences

When a woman is struggling to become pregnant, life develops a sense of being on hold. Her dreams and hopes for the imagined family feel less secure. She may be watching her friends have pregnancies and children. This emphasises her own childlessness and may create a feeling of isolation from those she was previously close to. Her job, often a refuge and place of success, may be providing less satisfaction, but she may be fearful of making changes just in case she becomes pregnant.

Most men want to become parents and hope to have children so they can encourage and engage them in the things they have enjoyed in life. But they perceive the future differently. Most men stay at work after having a child, so their work, activities and friendships do not change as much. Generally they expect to keep working while the woman is on parental leave, and they can look for advancement and change in their working lives without feeling compromised by the arrival of the child.

This does not mean that men do not feel sadness and loss with each period—they do, but generally it impacts less on their daily lives and their outlook for the future. Sometimes women feel that because men may not be shedding tears and expressing their sorrow they do not feel it. Men recognise the different experience for their woman and want to help her through this, but often want to support their partner by holding their own feelings to themselves. Women will say they are helped by knowing that men are feeling loss also. Open communication, both talking and listening, is important.

Loss of hopes and dreams

The initial loss begins as the hope and dream to become parents is not fulfilled. The desire to be pregnant and the fantasy about telling friends and family of the hoped-for child are not realised. The imagined family may be one of the woman or man's favourite dreams, and giving this up is challenging.

As time goes by, the couple face acknowledging they may have problems. Initially help may come through reading and looking for information on the web. Some couples try alternative therapies and only when they have had a lack of success do they consult the medical profession.

It may be hard to realise and accept that getting pregnant can take work and that other people will need to be involved for this to happen. The fear that it may never happen is too great to take on board, so the couple seek professional help to resolve the issue.

Seeking help

Sometimes people begin with their GP, although many self-refer to a fertility clinic. While waiting for an appointment with the fertility specialist, tests are done to provide information for the meeting. The couple may swing between anxiety and hope in this time. Anxiety because they may hear things they do not want to know, and hope that it may be a simple fix. For many couples the news they will need the clinic and a treatment programme to be able to parent may bring a sense of relief—at least they have a pathway. There will probably also be a sadness about needing other people involved in their baby-making.

The couple need to talk about how it feels for the woman to have invasive tests, for the man to have to produce a sperm sample in difficult circumstances, and the impact of receiving news both good and bad. Treatment involves a series of blood tests, scans and results, which are sometimes good news but can produce undesired outcomes and the sadness that accompanies this. Developing good communication early on equips people to deal with the process of treatment. By sharing these things with each other the couple are able to support each other and reduce the pressure the unknown brings with it. When a couple are about to undertake treatment they will cope best if they are relatively emotionally robust. Treatment may take some time to be successful, and can have times of excitement and hope as well as disappointment and sadness if the dream is not fulfilled.

Grief while receiving fertility treatment may be triggered by a poor response to the drugs, by the cycle not proceeding to its conclusion, by embryos not forming well, by a negative pregnancy test or when a result is positive but a miscarriage or biochemical pregnancy occurs (where there is an initial positive pregnancy test but the pregnancy does not progress). No one wants these things to happen, but being strong together will help both the man and the woman get through them.

Coping with grief and loss

Coping with loss and the sadness, fear, guilt, shame, unworthiness, resentment and myriad other feelings is a big task. Grief is a complex process. With infertility, each person deals with their own sense of loss while (if part of a couple) trying to support the person they love. If support does not come easily then it is a lonely time.

It is often difficult to seek support outside of the relationship as you may feel others do not understand. Your friends and family may love you, but they may not have had difficulties getting pregnant and even telling them may be hard. Often people do not tell their families because they are unsure about the family's capacity to deal sensitively and privately with their situation. The couple fear unsolicited advice, and even jokes, as family and friends struggle to cope with the information.

When the infertility comes from one person in the couple, this may make that person feel guilt and unworthiness in the relationship, and they may need a lot of reassurance and love to get through it. The other partner meanwhile may be feeling sadness and a level of resentment at having to go through the treatment when there is nothing wrong with them. We form stable relationships because we like and love each other—the relationship is not conditional on future fertility. Indeed relationships all have events happen in their lifespan and learning to deal with these together provides a strength for us.

Finding someone to talk with is often useful here. Some things are difficult to say to your partner because you know they may be hurt by them and not understand that they are part of what is going on for you.

Josh

Josh came to counselling by himself. He arrived looking fragile, with his emotions close to the surface. After reassurance of the confidentiality of the session he began to pour out the feelings and behaviours that he had been dealing with since seeing the fertility specialist the previous week.

He told me that he had found out that he did not produce sperm, and while the doctor would do some testing to see if they could find sperm, the doctor did not hold out much hope as Josh had a condition called Klinefelter syndrome. This is a random genetic anomaly that meant he had an extra X chromosome and probably low testosterone and no sperm.

Josh was devastated. He talked about not being a proper man, about not being worthy of the wonderful woman he had married. He feared his family's reaction and ridicule from friends. While he talked, his voice and words told of his sadness, disbelief and desperation to find a way through this.

He felt puzzled because he had no trouble ejaculating and satisfying his wife sexually—surely that meant he was a man? He was unsure what being a man meant now, and how he was going to manage in the future. His desperation and anger at this turn of events spilled out in tears and a raised voice as he tried to express these feelings.

Josh punctuated his story with 'Why me?', 'What have I done to deserve this?' and 'Will she stay with me?' It transpired that since the doctor's appointment Josh had put up a barrier between himself and his wife—refusing to talk, to cuddle, or allow any support for each other. It was only when he could not cope at work and they suggested he 'Get a counsellor and sort himself out' that he felt he should take action. His wife knew he was with the clinic counsellor and had offered to come, but accepted that Josh thought he should be by himself this time.

Much of this appointment was taken up by his need to express his emotions, and eventually he sagged in his seat and sat back and said, 'Help me, help us.'

Josh and I talked about his perception of their marriage before they went to the doctor's appointment. He told me of the love they had for each other and their joy in being together. His fear that he would lose this came from his belief that manliness was about making a baby.

We affirmed the need to grieve and that this grief would change over time. We talked about his learning to live with it. In an attempt to help him move forward we talked about things for him to think about. The first was why he and his wife had made a commitment to each other—was it about their love for each other or was it because they thought they would make good children together? Secondly we talked about manliness and where he got his ideas and fears from. Then we discussed how it must be for his wife when he would not talk with her and allow her to express her sadness about the situation and her continuing love for him.

Josh left wanting to talk about it with his wife and find ways to enjoy being together again. He also made an appointment for them to come to counselling together so they could be a team in dealing with the situation.

Most of our beliefs and values have been learned from childhood, from our families, and refined through our life experiences. We often do not think about beliefs and values until there is a reason to do so, such as when they are challenged. Josh had learned what manliness was as he grew up, and he had learned what challenged manliness.

He had also absorbed that he should not show his distress to his wife. Fortunately his work asked him to talk to a counsellor when his distress interfered with his work performance. Using a counsellor—a person who is only in your life for a set purpose—as a shortcut to understand the event, the feelings it produces, its impact on you, and strategies for coping is an effective means to help move forward.

The capacity to cope with loss is affected by a number of things—age, gender, experiences of prior losses, self-identity, support and the beliefs of those supporting us. Age and readiness to have children means, for most of us, that we have learned about loss and how to grieve. Few of us get to adulthood without losing a grandparent or a pet, shifting home or having a relationship end. Any of these and other experiences teach us that for the short time after the event it is hard to accept and that we may have poor control of our emotions. As time goes by our cognitive processes help us to make the plans necessary to have a funeral, to farewell a loved pet, or to have the appropriate response to another event. Additionally the world requires us to step back into our routine and begin functioning once again—getting back to work, and caring for each other and for the other people affected. While these things are going on the grieving person is finding a place in themselves to remember the event and cope with it as part of their life experiences. We do not forget losses that are worth grieving, but we do learn to live our lives and integrate that loss into our life. Loss and grief in infertility is different and generally goes on for a longer time.

The consent we give ourselves to grieve is important. Often societies allow the crying and wailing of a woman to release her emotions, but require of men a much more muted response. This does not mean men do not grieve; they are mostly just as effectual at grieving, but it is a different way of acknowledging the loss and supporting those around them.

Communication within the couple

When fertility is the loss and both people in a relationship are grieving, the acknowledgement of the loss to yourself and to each other is important. Often one person will make an assumption about how this is affecting their partner without checking with them. Talking about the loss with your partner helps you understand how this is for them, and it also allows the conversation to begin and to progress—this is of benefit as isolation occurs when we hold the feelings inside. Isolation can lead to withdrawal and a roadblock in communication. This will affect every aspect of your lives together.

Infertility is an invisible loss. When we are in the midst of it we may not realise the enormity of it, and if we keep it close others may not be aware of the impact it has on us. When we do not share our grief, others cannot offer the kindness and empathy that help us recover. Sharing grief allows us recognise and name the emotions, to work through them as we process what is happening. Talking and sharing helps speed up our processing of infertility.

Some people try to suppress grief by overeating, drinking or taking medication, others bury themselves in their work or withdraw from others. It is more useful to allow yourself to feel sad and accept the care and love of the important people in your life and so begin the acceptance of the situation. It means that if you decide to have treatment, you will be more emotionally able to cope with it. You can also prepare for it by becoming informed so you can make the decisions needed together. Feeling as if the decisions belong to both of you means you are more likely to feel involved through the treatment.

Managing grief and loss

From the time you acknowledge you need help, you become involved in another world—this test, that treatment, moving on to another type of treatment. The moving through treatment brings hope and often sadness. It's vital that you learn to care for yourself through the successive experiences, and to find ways that you can acknowledge each cycle, then manage your life so that the sadness—if it comes—does not overwhelm. As time goes by, your reaction to the experiences changes, often evolving as a result of your cognitive processes helping you to accept what is happening. Using cognitive parts of your mind stops the emotion overwhelming you.

Seeing yourself and your life through infertility alone diminishes you. We, as people, are so much more. We are members of families that love and care for us, we are workers who contribute to our workplace, we belong to cultures and beliefs that may provide a spirituality that supports us, we have friends and we do activities we enjoy. Somehow many of these things feel less valuable when we are facing infertility, yet it is these people and activities that keep us functioning well and help us resist becoming obsessive with the loss and grief of infertility.

There are things that you can do to keep a balance in your life. By reviewing your lifestyle and noticing change, you can remind yourself what helps you to be emotionally resilient (see 'Resilience in times of waiting'). Have you stopped doing activities that you've enjoyed in the past? Recognising if you've stopped going for regular walks or runs, if you're avoiding going out to movies or with friends, or if you're spending a lot more time at home, on your screen, is key. The things that have worked well to keep you engaged in life are worth keeping on with. Maybe they need small changes, but giving these things up completely creates a void, which can easily contribute to a feeling of depression.

Some of us will decide to do something new, perhaps finding a way to gain some success in activities—a new sport, learning a new activity, changing to another variation of an exercise programme, being creative in some way, DIY activities around the home. Others decide they will acknowledge each treatment cycle by an activity, a ritual, that becomes an ending for that cycle—this may involve writing about it and then putting the writing and results in a safe but out-of-the-way spot. One couple I worked with always went camping after a failed cycle—going back to nature and refreshing themselves by being among the bush, the birds and the beach. Seeking closure from a loss means you acknowledge the loss properly and are able to move forward.

Sometimes we get stuck and find it hard to do more than drag ourselves through the days. At this point we probably need to take a break from treatment and get some feeling of normal life back. This may be the time to evaluate the cost, especially emotionally, of the treatment and try to find ways that allow us to keep moving forward.

In New Zealand's bigger towns and cities there are support groups for infertile people—and the people who attend these meetings have experience and often understanding and strategies which may be useful to help manage the ongoing grief. If you cannot access a support group, look on Facebook and see if there is anything there that will help. Trying to stay within New Zealand sites when online will give you the best information and understanding.

Grief and loss when treatment ends

The end of treatment may come for a variety of reasons. There may be nothing more the clinic can offer, further treatments may be outside of your values (such as gamete donations), or you may simply have run out of emotional capacity to continue and want to regain some control of your life. Sometimes it is an economic decision to stop. Whatever the reason, at the end of treatment we face a life without children and need to be able to recreate a life that feels worthy, challenging and enjoyable.

When living this life, we acknowledge the loss of the children we had hoped for, and the future as we had always imagined it would be. We find other people and activities that make life of value. 'Chapter 20: Living without children', may provide some ideas.

Things to think about

- Grief is normal. It does not cause infertility; infertility causes grief.
- Feeling out of control is common. How can you manage it?
- Seeking help through information and advice gives back some sense of control.
- Are you sharing your feelings and valuing your relationship with your partner?
- Discuss who each of you tells among family and friends.
- Having support is helpful—women often need a confidante outside of the relationship.
- How much you tell someone else is a consideration. Once someone knows, you cannot change this.

Things that might be helpful

- Talking to each other and listening to each other is the best start to accepting the loss.

- Finding someone who understands this loss may help—this may be a support group, a Facebook group or the counsellor at your clinic.
- Friends and family can be helpful, but if they are fertile they may not understand the depth of the loss and, if treatment is not successful, the repeated losses. Often they will try to be helpful with suggestions. They have good intentions, but sometimes it is best to stay clear of the topic with them.
- Keeping up with activities that distract you and lower stress helps—exercise, yoga, mindfulness, reading, movies, etc.
- Work keeps structure in your day and a feeling of being successful, which can balance the failure to get pregnant.

Chapter 3

Self-esteem

Sarah and Allan

We began our quest for a child full of hope, with assumptions it would be easy and a strong sense of who we were both individually and as a couple. The continual arrival of periods began to concern us, and our response was to withdraw as a couple from our family and friends, who all seemed to think it was fine to ask when we thought we might have a family.

Our stress levels went up and our communication with each other went down. Our lovemaking became a task. Exercise was a way of filling in time and hoping to feel better. Our lives were ceasing to be those of happy individuals or a motivated couple.

These are frequent thoughts, feelings and behaviours for couples as they try unsuccessfully to create a child. With the strong interaction between the thoughts and the messages this couple was giving themselves, they were on the way to losing their self-confidence.

At this stage of attempting to have children it is common to research on the internet to try to ascertain why conception is not occurring. Some information may be useful, but much of it may cause further anxiety and confusion. Recognising the need to seek knowledgeable help through a medical professional is the beginning of accepting something may be wrong.

Maintaining a positive sense of self when faced with infertility is difficult. Part of this difficulty is that others can make having children seem easy. Another part is the long time it often takes to sort out the reason and find a solution. Protracted time to resolve infertility requires clear thinking. It needs emotional strength, resilience, effective communication, and access to resources, such as support.

Being gentle with yourself and your partner in thoughts and actions helps ease the pathway through this time. Blame and arguing undermine both of you, whereas having compassion and self-compassion leads to acceptance and self-care. One way of dealing with this is to ask yourself the question: 'How would I talk to a close friend in this situation?' Then apply the same words of comfort and understanding to yourself and your partner. By doing this you will feel better in yourself.

Infertility feels uncontrollable, unpredictable and stressful. These are all factors that affect our self-esteem and our sense of our self as a valuable person. Self-esteem can be thought of as the extent to which we prize, value, approve of and like ourselves. The desire to think of ourselves as valuable drives our behaviour and shapes the way we think. Among other things self-esteem has the function of helping maintain wellbeing, facilitating self-determination (having control of our life), reflecting on our status and providing information about inclusion or exclusion into desirable groups. These are all affected by infertility.

Understanding self-esteem

Self-esteem underpins everything we undertake, so enjoying life and feeling successful improves our self-esteem. It begins developing as soon as a baby is given attention by its parent(s) through such behaviours as feeding, comforting, holding, stroking and talking. These actions indicate to the child that he or she is lovable and has supportive people around. Children who are given this attention are more likely to have a positive sense of themselves (self-image and self-worth). As a result they are more likely to be able to problem-solve, and to accept making mistakes and not achieving all their goals. They will have positive internal dialogue or self-talk, which, along with a strong sense of identity, can help to answer questions such as 'Who am I?' and 'Do I need to make changes?'

Self-image is how a person sees themselves in the world. When our self-image is intact we are able to manage our lives and we feel we are of value. Self-image contributes to self-worth.

Not all people are lucky enough to grow up in a nurturing, caring environment, and some people will have changes in their lives as a child that mean care is less available. This may be through the stress of a parent, ill health or loss of a significant person.

Catching and then challenging thoughts that create a negative sense of self is important. When you find yourself having thoughts that catastrophise, such as *I will never become pregnant,* challenge this by asking yourself *How can I know this?* or saying *Never is a long time and I can't see that far.* By interrupting these negative thoughts with challenges, we save ourselves from slipping down.

Gaining a positive sense of self-worth and working to maintain this in the face of difficulties such as infertility requires a good level of self-knowledge and a capacity to recognise what is needed for the next step.

Anna

Anna's mother died when she was 15. Up until then she had received positive attention from her mother and believed she had a reasonable sense of herself. After her mother's death Anna went to live with her uncle's family—parents and four children with vastly different ways of communicating and behaving. She felt constantly put down and talked over, and her belongings became the whole family's property—she lost her sense of identity, autonomy and competence. Her need to grieve was not acknowledged, and sharing a room meant she had little privacy to recollect her mother and their life together. She temporarily lost her earlier childhood as her source for coping and making changes to her life.

Anna lived with her relatives for two years, struggling at school and silent at home. She made the decision at 17 that she needed to leave this home and create another life. In her last months with the family she began work in a fast-food outlet and gathered together resources so she could move into a flat with others and apply for tertiary education.

Life was better for Anna after she made these changes, and gradually she emerged with a more positive sense of herself. She formed a loving relationship with Gary.

When Anna was 27, she and Gary tried for children, and they eventually found their way to a fertility clinic. Anna was quick to access counselling as she felt a resurgence of the lack of self-worth she had felt after her mother died. The feelings belonging to her previous negative self-worth began to re-emerge, and she blamed herself for their difficulties in getting pregnant, despite the couple not knowing their issue. She knew that without help she would be likely to sabotage herself and her relationship.

Anna, and then Anna and Gary, had several counselling sessions in which they talked about the impact of Anna's past. They learned that the feelings she had in her mid-teens could be triggered by other situations where she felt out of control and unsure about herself. When prompted, Anna also remembered the feelings of love and worth she had had with her mother and now had with Gary. This understanding of feelings and of where they came from allowed Anna to separate her current experience from her tricky two years with her uncle and family. It allowed her to talk with Gary and for him to understand why she was vulnerable in this way. Together they made their way through the process of tests, diagnosis and treatment.

The specialist was unable to find a reason for Anna and Gary's lack of pregnancy and they chose to do an IVF cycle. They had a child from the first embryo and went on to have a second child.

The importance of understanding each other and communicating on a deeper level is important when issues around fertility arise. Couples will change as they experience a lack of success, and this will bring to the surface old frailties. The capacity to speak about them and to reduce the power of this old learning is significant. It helps stop us from undermining ourselves. Having your partner, a family member or a friend as an ally and understanding your and their feelings and how they have arisen is a potent tool. It allows us to operate as a team and create balance in the value of these experiences.

Self-esteem is the state of mind where we are able to appreciate or like ourselves. Self-esteem lets us monitor the way we feel valued as a partner in a relationship; it is part of self-evaluation. By having someone close to talk with and who is a good listener, it is possible to hear our self-assessment. This allows us to decide if this is what we want to be, and it allows change. This discussion requires trust and confidence in our listener.

With infertility, and especially for those people who are infertile, self-worth may take a tumble. Given that our feelings come from our thoughts and that both feelings and thoughts influence our behaviours, it is little wonder some people fall into a doldrum and need someone they can trust to help them out of it.

Jody

Jody sat, trying to stay calm, and said, 'How can I feel okay about myself when I can't even give my relationship a child? I have a faulty body. I am not truly a woman. I no longer feel attractive, sexual or even capable of running my life. What can I do to make it worthwhile being with my partner, to keep this person I love with me? Who wants a broken woman?'

These are strong feelings of despair and lack of self-worth. Feelings similar to this may be common fears for some infertile people. By finding someone she trusted and hearing herself talk about her feelings, Jody was able to think about them and was able to ask herself if these feelings were right. Jody recognised that the feelings had not existed yesterday and that what had changed was a piece of information she now had. She was able to take that further and realise that her partner had loved her yesterday and that it was her sense of not being lovable that was getting in the way.

Finding a way back through diminished self-esteem involves recalling what we liked about ourselves before the event—what we enjoyed doing, who we enjoyed being with, what we got a sense of success from. By identifying these factors and trying out some of the behaviours associated with them, the thoughts and feelings return. The positive feedback loop of feeling, behaviours and thoughts can be re-established.

Things to think about

- Everyone needs a level of support. Sometimes our partner is enough, sometimes we need more. If you feel very private, or your partner wants to keep it private, seek support from a professional such as the counsellor at the clinic. Support from a close friend or family member who will respect your confidentiality works well.

- You are the same person you were before you knew the information about your infertility, so try not to pass all your personal power to that piece of information. You can do this by continuing with the life you had before and distracting yourself from letting fertility issues dominate your days.
- Are you thinking clearly and planning so you don't get caught up in negative thoughts?
- Activities such as work or volunteering give you a feeling of success, and this helps to create a balance to your feeling of lack of success in getting pregnant.

Things that might be helpful

- Make a list of all the things you have enjoyed doing previously and try out some of these again.
- Maintain a level of exercise—it provides wellbeing. Moving physically also helps move the feelings (behaviours change feelings)

and helps encourage positive feelings.

- Try not to isolate yourself; still have time with friends and family—they care for you.
- Spend time with the people who support you, and if you choose to tell them they will try to understand.
- Be wary of advice. People are trying to help but may not be very informed.

Chapter 4

Beliefs and values—how these can help or hinder

We all come to adulthood with beliefs about the way the world works and how we can manage life. These beliefs come from our upbringing, significant people in our lives and our interactions or experiences with the world. Our values are formed often from our beliefs as we mature. They may be the values we are given by our families or they may evolve as we interact with others. For some of us the beliefs and values we espouse come from our religion or cultural beliefs.

From our beliefs and values come our attitudes to things and events—such as our willingness to undertake fertility treatment. Our behaviours are the external evidence of our beliefs, values and attitudes. These all influence us, and can be reviewed and accepted or changed if necessary.

A number of us who need fertility treatment have not thought about how treatment fits into our model of the world. We have not had to develop beliefs and values around having children through fertility treatment. It may take some time while we learn about the fertility process and talk with our significant family and friends before we are ready to undertake treatment. This is perfectly normal, as one of the assumptions most of us have is that we will be able to have children naturally when we are ready, and so it requires thought and consideration to accept fertility treatment as a pathway. Once treatment begins it requires involvement in the process—for example, activities such as injecting yourself with hormones are outside of normal behaviours.

Others will know their culture or beliefs can cope with some aspects of treatment but not others. For example, some religions can cope easily with fertility treatment until donor eggs or sperm are suggested—they see involving a third party as a step too far. There are some belief systems that inform people they should accept their infertility and find other ways of fulfilling their lives.

We each have a choice regarding how much the acceptance of our beliefs and values plays into using fertility treatment. For some, having children is so important that they find a way through the maze of beliefs and values and accept that science is part of God's plan and using this science is therefore condoned. For others, getting their heads around the science of the treatment is too hard, and so they decide to look at another way of parenting, such as adoption. Sometimes people initially refuse fertility treatment then change their minds and come back to explore it after they have had time looking into other options.

Danielle and Joseph

IVF is our only chance of having a child together—we don't have enough sperm to fertilise an egg any other way. Along with our families, we are Christians, and we belong to a church that is conservative in its values. We have not had to question where our faith stood on an issue until now.

When we were told IVF was our best option we went to ground for a while to think about whether we could consider this. The plan we developed was to talk first with family and then, if all thought it necessary, with our pastor. We called a family meeting and talked with them about IVF. This was a big task, as they had no knowledge at all about infertility or the treatment available.

Explaining it to them helped us to clarify and truly confirm that we wanted to be parents. Family were able to come on board with us. So with their help we decided it was okay to use this science.

At this point we have said okay to going on the government waiting list for IVF. We are still unsure how our church stands on the use of this science. The questions that we find too hard to ask the church at the moment are around creation of embryos in the laboratory. The church does not support termination of pregnancy, so how about creation of embryos in the lab? What happens if we have too many embryos? Is disposing of an embryo after our family is complete a form of termination? The problem is 'when does life begin?' We say that conception occurs when you make love and a baby, but what does that mean in the IVF world?

In our discussions at the clinic we have decided to make decisions based around the number of eggs we produce. If we have a single-figure number of eggs we will fertilise them all, but if there are more we will consider some of them being frozen as eggs. Eggs cannot produce a child, so that is easier in the decision-making. We are comfortable with this, and also if we get more children than the three we would ideally like, we can cope.

As with Danielle and Joseph, people need to gather as much information as possible so they can evaluate if there is a way they can feel comfortable with the combination of acceptance of the treatment and not denying their beliefs.

Assumptions and myths about fertility in our societies

Many people are shaken to the core when their assumptions about their fertility are challenged. Our societies in New Zealand have many myths and assumptions that are very unhelpful to those struggling to have children:

- All fertility issues are female-based. The reality is that about 40 per cent of problems lie with the woman, 40 per cent are male-centred issues, and the remaining 20 per cent involve both parties or the problem cannot be identified.
- Sadly some of the families and ethnicities in New Zealand are very patriarchal (male-led families). The men in these families will often not allow the woman to tell the truth

about why they are not getting pregnant, and so she assumes responsibility.

- The belief that 'if we work hard at an issue we will have success' is based on the work ethic that has existed for years. This is unhelpful if the woman has blocked tubes or the man few sperm, as no amount of work will get past these issues. Probably IVF will be required to get the eggs and sperm together.

- 'It is our God-given right to have children.' A portion of people who want children will not be able to have them. There are some issues that treatment cannot help. Some people will work through the options, such as using their own sperm and eggs, using donor sperm or eggs, checking the uterus and even moving to surrogacy, yet they are not successful. The cost of this, both emotionally and financially, may take years to accept and work through. Knowing where the 'line in the sand' exists for them is very important, as it allows people to plan to move forward and create a life that will provide challenge and pleasure in different ways.

- 'I still feel young, fit and healthy at 43, my eggs should be fine.' Staying fit and healthy is commendable and everyone should try to achieve that for themselves. Eggs unfortunately are affected by other things, such as a woman's aging. It is the DNA in the eggs that is affected by age. This means it is harder to achieve a pregnancy and there are more miscarriages. When women say their mother had her last child at 44, she has probably had several children and another pregnancy in her forties. It appears that pregnancy can protect eggs a little from the aging process.

- 'Life is only of value if we have children.' All people have times in their lives when they have satisfactory lifestyles that do not involve children. Remembering this and what was enjoyable and what made you feel valuable at other times is important, as this may provide clues to how you can continue with a good quality of life both through treatment and if ultimately unsuccessful.

Our child-based society

Most cultures and societies are focused around the family as the base unit. This means most aspects of life develop allowing for and often encouraging the presence of children. Public places and daily life in cafés and on the streets are geared to make it possible to take children to them. Consequently much of our conversation is focused around children.

Families celebrate the birth of a child or grandchildren multiple times—at baby showers, birth celebrations, naming parties and christenings, and the child's birthdays as they grow.

Society also has events and festivals that are largely family-and children-based: Easter, Christmas, Santa parades, Guy Fawkes, and times when there are holidays with schools shut and work closed so families can be together. These are often very tricky times for people wanting to have children.

For those who cannot or choose not to have children it seems other people do not have boundaries or sensitivity in questioning them about their intentions and then giving their point of view or advice.

Molly and Tom

Molly and Tom were really happy as a couple and did not feel the need to be parents. They both had jobs they were enjoying and achieving well in, and a lifestyle with friends who, like them, were without children. They received pressure from their families to produce a grandchild and, after nearly a decade of being a couple, thought they would have one child. They told their families they were thinking this, and they received caring but unwelcome comments about families with only one child.

Having a child turned out to be difficult. Molly was 39 and her AMH (the blood test that measures egg reserve in ovaries) was low; Tom had a poor sperm count, with low numbers and poor morphology (shape of the sperm and tails).

The couple then had to decide whether to go ahead with what they saw as quite intrusive treatment—they were going to need IVF, and the doctor had said the eggs would need ICSI to achieve fertilisation. They talked about their earlier wishes not to have a child and how this level of treatment felt as if it crossed their line of acceptance. They were also aware they had a 15 per cent chance of success and that that felt low. On the other side was the guilt they felt as family really wished them to have children and they knew the decision would cause grief for their families if they chose not to try for a child.

Molly and Tom struggled with their decision, and when they identified the impact the struggle was having on their relationship they decided to step back from trying to be parents and look after themselves as a couple. Once they had made this decision they commented on their sense of relief to know and be able to plan their future.

They were open with their families about the reasons for this choice and over time their families accepted their decision.

Being child-free, whether by choice or because there are no further acceptable options, requires courage. Almost every person I have met in this situation has been challenged about this decision, and has had to find a way to say firmly but respectfully that they do not wish to have this discussion. They usually have to say this multiple times and to many people.

Child-free people tend to be successful people who contribute to society in different forms. They form very strong, stable relationship bonds, have supportive family and friends, and often really enjoy their pets as part of their lives. They are interesting people who create a life that has been considered and involves successes in other areas such as work, interests and community involvement. They live well and feel as if they can make their decision of benefit to themselves and others.

Things to think about

- When is the time to tell the important people in your lives about what is happening for you?
- Who should you tell of your struggles? Perhaps only those who you want to know and who are supportive of you.
- Are you feeling an obligation to your families to produce children?
- Are you both on the same page about how far to go with investigations and treatment?
- Should you give yourselves permission to not attend that baby shower or family Christmas party when all the children will be there?

Things that may be helpful

- Enjoying your work and having success there.
- Taking on a new activity if you have time.
- Taking time after your fertility decision to care for yourselves.

- Using distracting activities—a good book or movie—when you are feeling a bit glum.
- Not engaging in unwelcome talk or advice—kindly telling people you do not want to have this discussion.
- Being with people who support you.

Chapter 5

Spirituality and emotional wellbeing

We are all so different and there is no 'one size fits all'. Our differences are in gender identification, appearance, beliefs, values and culture. These things all contribute to our understanding of spirituality.

Spirituality includes a sense of connection to something bigger than ourselves, and often involves our concept of the meaning of life. Being spiritual is a universal experience that involves us all. Even if we choose not to recognise it or do not like the words. We need meaning in our lives.

The difference between spirituality and religion is the degree of organisation of beliefs and practices in religion. These are usually shared by a group. Religion is about spirituality but with the beliefs of others supporting each person. Religion generally embraces spirituality as part of its practice. Spirituality is more often individual and has to do with making a sense of peace and purpose.

It does not matter how a person feels about the concept of spirituality, most people have a sense of their own spirituality. Whether people get this through nature, the bush or the sea, through being involved in their community, or through their culture or their beliefs, most people have a sense of what is important to them and how they value it and want to contribute to it. A spiritual person cares about themselves and is loving to themselves and others. They know their wellness will enable them to be part of the community of people to whom they wish to belong. Spiritual people tend to have positive relationships and high self-esteem, are mainly optimistic, and have a meaning and purpose in life. Spiritual people cope better in adversity.

Spirituality is likely to be culturally dictated. We learn our values and beliefs from our culture, and these may stay with us subconsciously or by consciously considering them and enhancing them. Some choose to reject them in their lives.

Some people will talk about their spirituality as having developed from their culture, others their love of people or the environment and commitment to wanting to care for others and the world.

Sara and Ant

Throughout their time together whenever Sara and Ant felt fragile and unconnected to their spirituality, they went to their bach on the Coromandel Peninsula. Being in the bush and in or by the sea allowed them to calm and ground themselves. Sara used creative visualisations of their precious place when she felt a need to ground herself but was unable to travel to their bach.

A knowledge of and sense of your own spirituality provides a strong foundation to help resource you when you are working through fertility issues. There is a lot of comfort in knowing that while this very difficult experience is happening you, the world around you is helping to care for and support you.

Te whare tapa whā

Te whare tapa whā is the model of wellbeing developed by Sir Mason Durie in 1982 from his beliefs and knowledge of Māori wellbeing. Te whare tapa whā likens our bodies' wellbeing to that of the wharenui or meeting house of Māori.

The wharenui has four equal and strong walls. Each wall represents an aspect of health, and as a home it needs four walls to stand up firmly. When one wall is challenged, the others help it by supporting it; they all work together. The walls of te whare tapa whā represent the four things that each person needs to be a fully healthy person: taha wairua, or spiritual wellbeing; taha hinengaro, or mental wellbeing; taha tinana, or physical wellbeing; and taha whānau, or family and social wellbeing. The connection to the whenua, land, forms the foundation.

When Māori are thinking about taha wairua they are exploring their relationship with the environment, their people and their heritage in the past, present and future.

The way people view wairua can be very different. Perhaps wairua is the capacity for faith or religious beliefs or having a belief in a higher power. Others may describe wairua as an internal connection to the universe. There is no right or wrong way to think of or experience wairua, but it is an important part of our mental wellbeing.

Within this model, spiritual essence is mauri or life force—it is who and what you are, where you have come from and where you are going.

There is a lot of wisdom within Māori culture and beliefs. Thinking in terms of good health and fertility, recognising the interconnection of the various parts of health and wellbeing aids fertility wellbeing. If a person or couple recognise that one part, say taha hinengaro, or mental wellbeing, is being affected by the diagnosis and treatment of infertility, they can ensure wellness in the other aspects, which may help them get through this period. If people choose to be private about their fertility issues, then taha whānau cannot care for them and they will need the other three aspects functioning well.

The relationship of spirituality to fertility

When we enter the world of compromised fertility we are generally well people who, like all people, have a few thoughts and doubts but are functioning competently in most aspects of our lives. The hiccup is that we are not getting pregnant.

When we find some part of ourselves is not working as it should be, our sense of self, both physically and mentally, is challenged. There may be an answer to overcome this problem, but we need to accept and work with this solution to maintain our emotional and mental health. Maintaining the other aspects of wellbeing, as mentioned under the heading 'Te whare tapa whā' above, supports us as we move through the journey.

Ted and Delia

Ted and Delia were living their lives comfortably and without children when Delia read a magazine discussing age and fertility. She showed the article to Ted and they talked about this for some time. They intended to have children but had not begun to try to conceive. These are thoughtful people who considered change and liked to be prepared. Guided by their naturopath they began with a detox to rid their bodies of any issues that could be detrimental to pregnancy. They also began to get fitter and to source all their food organically. They reduced their alcohol intake significantly and stopped consuming caffeine.

Feeling well prepared, they spent six months trying to become pregnant. Then they saw the doctor at the fertility clinic, who felt Delia's ovulation was compromised and decided they might need a drug to stimulate ovulation. This drug caused Delia to become emotional and to feel out of control. She doubted herself, and quickly Ted became concerned.

On good advice they decided to deal with the panic that washed over Delia sometimes, and to do this by practising mindfulness.

Mindfulness worked well for them and Delia started to recognise she had tools to help her through this experience—tools such as using her breathing, when she began to feel anxious, to quieten the anxiety. Life became more settled, although they decided on their specialist's advice to change the stimulation drug to one that affected Delia much less.

She and Ted were unsure whether it was the mindfulness and being in touch with themselves that worked, or the new drugs. It was with joy that they learned they had conceived. Mindfulness continued to play a large part in their lives and wellbeing.

When we are supported by our beliefs and our sense of ourselves and where we fit in the world, this support will help us cope with our fertility problems. The strength we can gain from knowing who we are and accepting ourselves as functioning in most aspects of our lives supports and balances the sadness and disappointment that we feel in having a fertility issue.

This is important, as the treatment begins when women take fertility drugs or men have further testing. What is happening may feel invasive and compromise our sense of ourselves as a competent person. Being able to go back to who we think we are and how we fit in the world helps provide strength to continue.

Enhancing wellbeing

Wellbeing is a state that we tend to take most notice of when we are not feeling as good as we like to feel. Maybe something such as fertility challenges begin to consume our thoughts and we change some of the activities we normally do that take care of us.

Thinking about what is important to you, including what you value and wish to retain in your life, allows you to ensure you are true to yourself. For instance, if you have always enjoyed your picnics as you explore the areas around you, keeping enjoying these activities will help in your wellbeing.

Life is not always smooth for any of us, but having tools that allow you to keep some balance in your life when one aspect gets tough is important. Balance helps make sure that no one aspect of your life dominates and causes other useful aspects to be forgotten. Balance is about having some control over your thoughts and activities and catching yourself when you are getting out of balance. It is also about being kind to yourself and taking care of yourself. So if your thoughts begin to be dominated by your fertility treatment and the results of tests and scans, make sure you make time in each day for activities that distract you from these thoughts.

Motivation may be an issue in getting going with other activities. Knowing that exercise really helps us feel better is different from finding the capacity to get going on some exercise. At times like this the best question is: 'What would help me get going?' Maybe you need your partner or a friend to come with you, maybe just being kind to your dog will help you get out for a walk, maybe you can listen to music on your headphones while you walk to reduce your thoughts. There are many things we can do to change the nature of exercise and make it easier to undertake. Sometimes an alternative activity—gardening, DIY, or creative projects—will work well.

Everyone knows that taking care of physical health is important for fertility, for example ensuring you eat well, with lots of fresh vegetables for trace elements, not having too many takeaways, limiting your intake of caffeine and alcohol, stopping smoking, vaping and recreational drug use, and getting exercise. These givens make a difference and are things we can control as we have fertility treatment.

Our mental wellbeing is also important, and often a more difficult field to ensure wellbeing. When we feel down it is important to remember the things that give us joy, and often having a brainstorm and writing down the things that have given us joy is helpful. Staying connected with the people we love and are supported by is helpful. These are the people who will listen and talk about issues with us. They continue to love us even when we are having a tough time.

One recognised activity for creating happiness is doing voluntary activities. Giving to others allows us to feel we are contributing to our world and not just taking. People who give to others have higher happiness levels—the giving may be of time, listening or doing things for others. Giving helps us to stay connected and to recognise that everyone has needs, and by being in contact with others and their needs we can keep our own in perspective. Noticing change in others, our gardens, the weather and the seasons means we are looking outwards and being less self-occupied. This is a sign we are working well on our mental wellbeing.

As in maintaining our mental health, our family, whānau and friends are important in our wellbeing. Often the people who have known you all of your life are able to wrap unconditional love around you. They may need to learn what it is you need, but they are willing to keep loving you through this difficult period. Not everyone receives the support they need from their family; they may receive only the support their family is able to give. When this is not enough or the right type of support, then reaching out to wider family or friends is helpful.

Finally, understanding who you are and how you fit into the world is important. We all have many roles—as a daughter or son, a brother or sister, a partner, an employee or employer, member of groups or teams, friend to others, carer of pets, home and garden. All our roles are important, and most will not change as we seek to become parents. We need to value our roles and in doing that value ourselves.

Things to think about

- Does your life have a balance that supports you in coping during your fertility treatment?
- Are you caring for your physical self adequately? What might be a good change?

- Who are your support people that you can talk with when things are tough?
- What activities give you a sense of pleasure and positive wellbeing?
- How are you reaching out to be aware of others' needs and to care for them?

Things that might be helpful

- Taking the opportunity with your partner or a friend to review life as it is. Do you have balance, what has slipped, how can you change things, how will you know if you are doing better?
- Thinking about and acknowledging the small things that went well, at the end of every day.
- Seeking someone to talk with.
- Looking out to others in your world and listening to them and their stories. Try to reduce the focus on you and your infertility.

Chapter 6

The waiting game

Waiting is such an ordinary word, but it is one most fertility clients learn to dread. Everything takes time, and there is so little any person can do to feel they have control over the time. From the time we think about beginning a child, time feels elongated and becomes either a time of hope or a time of sadness.

Each month we wait and hope our period will not arrive, and if it does we begin again to try with the next month. The months add up and we begin to doubt whether we will ever become parents. The impact of waiting begins as a gnawing anxiety, and it fleshes out to a need to do something other than just keep trying. Our beliefs and assumptions about the future look shaky and that does not feel good. We can try to ignore this feeling, but that is difficult. This not-good feeling begins to challenge some of the things we value about ourselves.

Liam and Jamie

We—me and Jamie—have been together since we were at school. From day dot we talked about how lucky we were to find each other early. We decided from the beginning to spend our lives together—growing up, getting educated and getting good jobs, finding a home and all that. We had both grown up in families that had no spare anything and we did not want that. We just wanted to get sorted out so we could settle.

We followed our plan and I became an electrician earning good money; Jamie as a nurse also earned well, so we bought a home—not fancy, but comfortable.

Now was the time to have children—mid-twenties and set up. We were so proud, and had a ceremony as we put away the contraceptive pills and began life making love to make a baby instead of just because we loved each other. We knew it might take around six months to get pregnant while Jamie's body adjusted to life without the pill, so were not concerned when her periods arrived, just a bit disappointed.

After six months Jamie began reading about why we might not be getting pregnant—so many possible causes. She went online and looked at the local fertility clinic information and decided we should see a specialist. We got an appointment, did the tests and went to see the doctor. She was very nice, but could not give us any reason for either of us to explain why this was not happening.

We were not eligible for government funding as we had not been trying long enough—for unexplained infertility we had to try for five years. This felt like forever. The doctor suggested we try a drug that would give Jamie's ovulation a little boost, but we needed to be aware that we ran the risk of twins if she produced two eggs and they both fertilised.

We decided to follow that path, and for four months Jamie took the pills and felt very emotional. We had sex at the right time of the month;

it was not really making love as it felt like a job.

This quickly became hell for us. We were bickering and finding fault with all the little things in life. We barely talked nicely together, and I began working longer hours as I dreaded seeing Jamie so out of sorts.

One night Jamie, in tears as she often was, said she could not carry on with this. She just wanted to be us again and to like being together. I was so glad when she said that.

So came a huge change for us. She stopped the pills, we planned a weekend away together and we got a puppy, which we had been delaying until we had a baby growing. Jamie took a month of leave without pay, I kept my work to eight hours a day, and we were careful in our communication together. We were both so glad to find ourselves again.

'Where to now' was something we talked about a lot, and since we were still under 30 we took our time considering.

We looked at the fertility clinic information and their statistics for success, then the cost of treatment, and decided we would move straight to IVF, which we would fund ourselves. Such a lot of money, but we didn't know how much treatment we could cope with so we decided to begin where there was the biggest chance of success.

Surprisingly Jamie had no trouble with the IVF drugs and we got 10 eggs and six blastocyst embryos. One replaced in the uterus and five frozen—great news.

This is such a waiting game. We had waited for six months before going to the clinic, we waited nearly six weeks to see a doctor, we tried over five months with the egg-stimulation drug, then waited for a couple of months before we went back to the doctor for a review and plan for IVF—then another couple of months before we started. This had all taken about 18 months. IVF has its own times of waiting—to see how many eggs we would get, then the tension-filled days to see how many became nice embryos.

And here we are today having an embryo transferred to Jamie's womb and then another nine long days' wait. So much waiting!

PS (a couple of years later): The first embryo took; we were lucky. We still don't know why we did not get pregnant ourselves, but our second child we started by ourselves—what a surprise—and now we are back on the pill!

Liam and Jamie felt they did a lot of waiting yet they got through the process relatively quickly, especially as they were able to pay for treatment. For many couples the wait is much longer.

A few lucky people get pregnant when they first wish to; most have a wait to conceive. Knowing when to stop trying to conceive by themselves and go to a fertility clinic for help is one dilemma facing those trying to get pregnant. Infertility is defined as having unprotected intercourse for one year and not conceiving. Yet it is commonly believed that people under 30 should conceive in about six months and that people over 35 should get going with treatment before their good fertility window starts to close. For these groups a time of six months is recommended.

It often takes time to get pregnant even with treatment. When the circumstances are not especially good for one or both partners it may mean trying more than one treatment. This can elongate the process significantly.

Lizzie and Harry

Lizzie and Harry finally went to the clinic after trying to get pregnant by themselves for a couple of years. The doctor told them they both had low-level fertility issues—Lizzie had low egg reserves in her ovaries, and Harry's sperm was a bit unusual in shape.

The doctor recommended IVF and put them on the Ministry of Health funding list. The wait was about 18 months. During this time they both took supplements recommended by the doctor and looked at the lifestyle issues relevant to them.

Finally they reached the top of the list and were able to try IVF. By this time Lizzie was 36 and Harry 35, so they were keen to get going.

Their first IVF produced only two eggs, neither of which grew into surviving embryos so they did not have an embryo replacement. They then had another cycle with a different IVF plan (longer cycle with more and different drugs) to try to get more and better-quality eggs. This time they got five eggs, and at day five there was a blastocyst to replace. Although desperately hoping for success they were unsurprised when they received a negative result.

The doctor's review suggested they should focus on finding an egg donor, and recommended the counsellor as the person who could help them learn about this.

Harry and Lizzie had now been trying for a baby for nearly five years and they realised it would be another couple of years (if they were lucky) before they would have a baby in their arms. Trying to become parents had dominated a large section of their adult life and time together.

Lizzie asked her younger sister Janie to donate eggs, and was delighted when she agreed. Her sister was breastfeeding and wanted to do this for another three months—she had fed her other child until one year old. They agreed Janie would start the process of seeing the doctor while still feeding. The doctor did tell them Janie would need a period after she stopped feeding before the IVF. Another wait for Lizzie and Harry.

It was a year after Lizzie and Harry's IVF that Janie provided them with 10 eggs, which resulted in three good-quality embryos. They were pregnant with the first, and hoped they may have another child.

Lizzie and Harry had seven years between beginning to try to conceive and having a child. Lizzie was almost 39 as a new parent, and she reflected she had given up a lot of life in the effort to become a parent. She had become preoccupied with her wish to become a parent and had become distant with most of her friends and ceased her interests and activities. Her recommendation to others in this situation is for them to ensure they have a better balance of activities in life than she managed.

While there are some people who will succeed with treatment quickly, for a good number the journey is long and often hard. The lack of success can take many forms, and each time something does not work another different pathway may be offered. There is always a wait to start a new treatment or to move to something new, like using a donor or surrogacy. This cycle of raising new hope and then despair can be very wearing for people.

The impact of waiting

Waiting to have a child can be a long and difficult experience, and the waiting involved in fertility treatment can also feel long. In treatment the times can be broken into smaller times of waiting—for drugs to work, for blood tests and scans and results, to see if embryos develop, for pregnancy, and maybe for the time to pass so we can begin again. All of this waiting can feel overwhelming, as if it takes over our lives.

The impact of successive periods of waiting can be big. Understanding the reason for the wait and the approximate likely length of the wait helps. As fertility investigations take place and the waiting periods for the results or for government funding go on, life often goes on hold. Some people stop many of the activities that had supported their sense of self and contributed to their wellbeing. Yet by ensuring you maintain your lifestyle, it is possible to reduce the impact of waiting. The activities that are vulnerable to being dropped are exercise, outings or coffees with friends, creative or DIY activities, and the general desire to initiate fun.

When we reduce these events our satisfaction with life lowers, as does our sense of self as a worthwhile person. The loss of self-belief when you cannot create a child as easily as friends or family have can permeate a lot of aspects of life.

By changing the frequency of involvement in lifestyle activities we risk our feeling of wellbeing. We isolate ourselves from those who are important and able to provide support. We lose our goals for the future and lose some of ourselves unless we are able to re-engage with life.

Maintaining wellbeing

Being aware of the ways that daily or regular activities contribute to a sense of wellbeing is important. If you like gardening, seeing the difference your efforts make gives a sense of success. If you enjoy a walk, the fresh air and endorphins from the exercise are helpful. Cuddling a pet, doing baking, building or mending something, or even playing a computer game can all give a sense of achievement. These activities in balance with other aspects of life such as work help to keep life in balance, especially when waiting for the next stage in fertility treatment.

Dissatisfaction with an aspect of life can be magnified when other parts of life, such as becoming pregnant, are not happening. A common area of discontent, especially for women, is their work. They have often stayed in a job that they are not really enjoying because they see parental leave as the way out of it. When a pregnancy does not eventuate, they focus on the job and may develop a sense of wondering if this is their lot in life. Making change can feel very difficult. Yet having choices is important and can give you back a sense of control. Considering options to maybe change jobs or retrain is useful when the fertility journey is taking longer than expected. Sometimes there are options such as a decision to make change within the current workplace; at other times retraining or changing employment is a better choice.

Finding the motivation

Having in focus the good things that give us enjoyment and feelings of success are important in helping us with the balance of life. Yet often the motivation to get into the garden and get things sorted or to get out for a walk or run is just too hard to muster. The activities we are challenged by are often the ones that act as stress-reducers in our lives. Finding a way to use them for wellbeing is important.

Waiting causes a lowering of mood. It is this feeling of being down that has to be overcome. Making the challenge smaller or getting a friend to join us in the activity often helps us get going. The satisfaction of completing even that smaller task is likely to help you the next time you begin the activity.

Achieving some satisfaction and success reduces the feeling of failure and loss of control. By succeeding in a small action, motivation can increase to help us do other good things with life. Success often leads to further achievement.

Motivation provides the energy for us to achieve a task and this lifts the mood. Getting started provides the motivation to keep going, enhancing the feel-good factor. A good example is going for a walk—beginning reluctantly but giving it a go means that after a short period the body, muscles and joints will loosen up and, as our body starts to feel easier, our mind and spirit will lift with it. Not only does the exercise provide physical and emotional benefit for us, we are also likely to feel positive about managing to get going. Some days this is harder than others, but taking the first step will help take the next step, and so on.

Procrastination has completely the opposite effect—by deciding not to do something most people will trigger the 'I should have...' script. This can lead to self-blame. This negative cycle needs to be broken before it spreads to other aspects of life.

In fertility treatment, with all the uncertainty and waiting, maintaining a positive lifestyle is one of the biggest supports we can give ourselves. This involves using the waiting time productively so we feel in good physical and emotional condition when the treatment begins.

A positive lifestyle

Many people are in a very good stage of life when they begin to think about becoming parents. They may have jobs they enjoy—jobs they are challenged by and that give a sense of competence. They may have a group of friends with whom they do activities and have fun. They may have their economic situation generally sorted and be aware that with parental leave they, or one of them, can have time off with their baby while it is young. They probably have plenty of support and care around them.

These people are likely to be engaged in activities that provide interest, commitment and challenge to their lives. This may be about their physical wellbeing, involvement with creative tasks, being social for recreation, or being with family and friends. For many people their spiritual wellbeing is part of this, whether it is through their religion, cultural beliefs or being engaged in nature, or other ways that people choose to look after their wellbeing.

All of these aspects of life provide pleasure, reinforcement and action. They can be sources of strength and support when life becomes tough to get through.

Resilience in times of waiting

Resilience is the capacity to cope with hurdles and recover quickly. We can work towards being resilient people by understanding which activities and people contribute to our coping well with life. Knowing ourselves and being able to move positively *before* we feel down are important strategies in life. Recognising that waiting for the next event in fertility is taxing and putting resilience strategies into practice really pays off.

Maintaining resilience can be tricky. Fertility treatment and the feelings of lack of control it produces can feel overwhelming. Understanding what supports you can allow you to care for yourself even when it feels there is no control of what happens, when it happens, or the outcome. Resilience is knowing what mechanisms work for you when there are setbacks or obstacles to success. It is about recovering after a setback and finding the confidence to go forward and sometimes to take another risk.

Being resilient involves having the self-knowledge to recognise stress and the strategies to cope with it. If the stressor is all the waiting, resilience means having activities and people in your life that will help you get through it and come out the other side.

On their website, which has many helpful resources designed to share, the New Zealand Institute of Wellbeing and Resilience talks of things that help.

1. Choose where you focus your attention—notice what's good in your world.
2. Deliberately seek out people and things you like to do that make you happier.
3. Nourish your relationships—strong supportive relationships are a good predictor of wellbeing.
4. Keep to daily routines or create new ones—live as normally as possible.

5.   Focus on what matters and what you can influence or control.

Recognising that waiting is stressful but inevitable, and working out how to best manage your waiting time, will improve your experience of fertility treatment.

Things to think about

- Who can you talk with and get fertility advice from?
- How long should you wait before seeking specialist help?
- What activities and which people help you to feel good?
- If one of you needs to confide outside of the relationship, how will you manage this, and what is okay to talk about?
- What are the activities that you do together that help you problem-solve?
- Are you treating each other with care and respect?
- What can you do to help your partner when they are down, and vice versa?

Things that might be helpful

- Talking openly and honestly, but being sensible and limiting the time spent talking about fertility so it does not take over your lives.
- Making a list of the activities you enjoyed prior to having fertility issues and keeping it handy—stuck up on the inside of a frequently used cupboard is good. When you are feeling a bit down, do something on the list to get yourself going.
- Keeping a calendar of appointments and things to do so you do not have to remember it all.
- Asking good questions of the fertility staff you are dealing with—about time waiting, about treatment. Often taking a list with you helps.
- If you are a very private person who does not wish to discuss things with people you know, or if you just think it would help, use the counsellor.

Chapter 7

Thinking about treatment

Fertility treatment has had a lot of publicity over the past two decades and most people of fertile age will either know someone or know of someone who has had IVF. Many of the people who have successfully had a child through IVF are happy to talk about it in an appropriate situation. Some people are happy to have publicity about their issues in the hope this will encourage others to seek help.

When you are told of the need for treatment it is often a very confusing time. While you hope for a solution, the reality that you need intervention presents you with a level of fear and uncertainty about what this means. You may have little or no knowledge of the treatment and need time and education to understand and come to terms with what is ahead. You need to consider how and with whom you can access time to discuss the treatment and its impacts. Talking with the clinic nurse will help you to learn about and understand the fertility treatment the doctor is recommending for you. Counsellors are able to break down the medical and scientific information into easy-to-understand language and can help resolve fears about treatment.

It is easy to find yourself focusing on the treatment to the exclusion of everything else in your life. Developing a balance between thinking about and preparing for treatment and distracting yourself so you can carry on with life is tricky.

Some people like to live their lives with as little medical intervention as possible. When they become aware of the need for technology, it is a big step for them to come to terms with, and sometimes a step too far. Even with a chance to discuss the treatment in depth and to help them understand it, they may struggle. They may need to talk with their specialist about whether they can begin with a less invasive treatment first. This may not be possible or worthwhile, but asking helps.

At the first interview with the doctor, the couple will be told either what the doctor has found or if there is a need for further testing to sort out what is going on. The shock of being told by the doctor they need treatment sometimes means they hear only fragments of the remaining information given to them. Often the couple will see their nurse after the doctor, and she or he may be able to help them understand and sort out which information they should read. Taking time to read, to think and to talk about the treatment helps a couple to consider what this will be like for them. Most clinics provide an accessible booklet or have an online site full of information to give to the client; in addition, the clinics' websites are easy to follow.

Shelley and James

We arrived at the clinic and suddenly felt overwhelmed by all the people sitting waiting and the staff looking so business-like. We gave our names to the receptionist and slunk into the furthest corner to just watch and to stop the pounding in our chests. If the lifts had not been just in front of reception, we probably would have sneaked out.

Our names were called. We looked over to see a youngish man in a shirt and tie looking our way. He was smiling ... Perhaps we could manage this.

We followed him into his office, and he showed us where to sit, then introduced himself. He seemed quite pleasant as he told us that today we were going to talk about the tests we had done and where we needed to go from there. So far it was good.

He began with me (Shelley), and said that I did not seem to be ovulating. I must have looked blank, so he explained that the blood tests I had done showed my body had not produced an egg that month, and in fact may not be able to produce eggs by itself. I was stunned and tearful, and the only thing I was aware of was James holding my hand tightly.

The doctor went and got us some water and then said he also had other things to talk about. He commented that he would like to do an ultrasound scan on me that day, as he suspected I had polycystic ovaries. I had heard of this, and had read they were one of the reasons some women found it hard to lose weight. I knew I was of the bigger size.

James, he told us, had slightly low sperm numbers, and he thought some lifestyle changes might help that. He asked James about smoking, drinking and recreational drugs. He suggested stopping smoking and recreational drugs and cutting back on alcohol, and that, while doing this, James should also take a fertility multivitamin. Apparently, it takes 10 weeks for new sperm to form, and by then he would have formed a new habit.

His nurse came in and they did the ultrasound, and it was confirmed I had polycystic ovaries. The doctor suggested some more tests and talked about losing some weight.

The doctor was really nice and we could understand him easily, but what we were told was all new to us and seemed so much to take in. We walked out in a daze, with blood forms and a book to read. We had hoped there was nothing wrong; instead we needed to make some hard changes in our lives. And we needed to do this before we could be scored for government funding for the treatment we were likely to need.

It took us about a week before we accepted what he had told us and were able to do the reading we were given. The changes we had to make are hard things to change, and it took us a long time to find a plan to change them. Eventually we went back for a review—I was 5kg lighter and James was not smoking or doing pot. The doctor had both our new results and we talked about IVF treatment. He put us on the list for government-funded treatment, which was pleasing. We asked for something not too complex first, and decided to try a drug to stimulate ovulation. We could afford to pay for this while we waited for our name to come up the waiting list for IVF.

It was amazing how much easier the appointment was this time. We had questions ready and could talk without bursting into tears. We felt as if we were definitely making progress and that in some way we would get a baby.

Many couples will need this time to process the potential treatment information and come to terms with what is required. There are other couples for whom there is no issue with treatment and who wish to begin straight away. Regardless, to avoid frustration people need to understand the purpose of further testing and delays.

If you are reliant on receiving government-funded treatment, the waiting time, which is often around 18 months, can seem long and sometimes unfair. Using this time to enhance the possibility of treatment being successful is the best strategy in this situation. This is the time to review your lifestyle and optimise it before beginning treatment. It is also a good time to take charge of stress levels so when you have treatment you do not have too many life challenges to deal with at the same time.

Cultural issues

Each clinic helps a range of different ethnicities, and hopes to fulfill their dreams if it is possible. The clinics try to be respectful of the needs of each ethnicity, and are open to people guiding them on their needs as long as it does not compromise the service they provide. For example, whānau from any culture are welcome. Most often they come to support our Māori or Pasifika people, and sometimes those from the Middle East. They are welcome to be alongside the patients and attend most appointments. When it comes to an egg collection, however, there isn't room in the theatres for more than one support person, and that is usually the partner or closest person.

Other ethnicities have different issues to deal with. Sometimes it is inappropriate for women to have male doctors conduct examinations. In such cases, female doctors can be made available. Another difference may occur when cultural beliefs and the Human Assisted Reproductive Technology (HART) Act, under which we work, differ. An example of this often occurs with donations. When the recipient couple need a donor to become parents, they may believe their family will not accept the child unless it is fully related to them. The couple may wish to keep the donation secret. The HART Act states clearly that each child has a right to their genetic information. The pathway through this is tricky, and the couple may need help to manage this.

It is not for me, as a Pākehā author, to state what Māori or other cultures need within the clinic. But I am aware that the clinics will support cultural needs as much as they are able. I would encourage people to find someone to talk with about practices and find a process that they both feel comfortable with. Examples of common issues I have seen in the clinic follow.

For many Māori clients, dealing with fertility issues happens within a clinic that essentially represents Pākehā medicine and culture. While some will feel comfortable as most of their medical experience happens in largely Pākehābased clinics, others will feel a level of shyness and sometimes shame about having to discuss such personal aspects of their lives with others. To be given advice, such as needing to lose weight before receiving funding or to change lifestyle habits, which would make them different from their network, is very challenging. There may be little support for them to do this in their lives.

Māori clients may be more comfortable if they have whānau with them for support. Clinics understand the need for whānau support and encourage Māori clients to bring their whānau.

While many Māori patients wish to just pass through the treatment process and get it over, there are some who wish to have a karakia or prayer said at stages of the treatment. They can request this opportunity and discuss how this best be managed. Clinics will do their best to accommodate requests like this.

TJ and Mala

TJ wrote of the sadness he and Mala felt when they could not become pregnant. The doctor told them he had found Mala had low ovarian reserve. TJ described he and Mala as a shy couple who could not ask family for help at that stage.

The clinic had one Māori egg donor available and so they all agreed to swap profiles and, if that worked, to meet. This all went remarkably well, and the couples—TJ and Mala and the donor and her partner—decided to do the IVF together. It was a success, and before the embryo replacement TJ asked if they could all come in earlier and have a private room so they could have a small ceremony. TJ welcomed the donor couple into their whānau, said a karakia and sang a waiata. It was a profound time for all—a joining not only through the sharing of an egg, but also an emotional and spiritual joining. They reshaped their families.

They have kept a close relationship, and the children of both families will know of the genetic connection. The donor couple are included in all activities on TJ and Mala's marae and in their family.

Commonly, the ethnicities other than Māori and Pākehā who attend the clinics are Pasifika, Asian, Indian and Middle Eastern. Each of these brings their own needs, such as privacy, dealing with a specific gender of doctor, and language issues. Ensuring clinics are told about the patient's needs means they will endeavour to accommodate them. Interpreters are available with some notice. The doctor's nurse, who is generally very accessible, will do their best to help people to feel as comfortable as possible.

English as a second language

As difficult as it is finding a pathway through the treatment and technology, for people who speak a different first language it is even more difficult.

Patients who have English as a second language may need to seek further support to understand the information. There are a number of options for this. Taking along a competent English speaker as a support person who can listen and ask questions or discuss what was heard later is very useful. This support person may also be able to help you read and understand the handbook.

Many people who are not easy English speakers prefer to use an interpreter. Clinics are able to organise this on request.

Different cultures have different needs and ways of interacting. It adds an extra level of difficulty if the way you hear and interpret behaviours and words is different from the professional who is talking to you. The process of medical appointments is defined, and people often feel this means they are not getting personalised treatment and the understanding they need. The language and experience barrier may make people feel as if they are not being as well looked after as they would wish. It is important to let the clinic know about the situation and they will attempt to sort out the issue. The general solution to this is to get an interpreter who will not only help your understanding, but will also explain to the health professional how this is for you.

Infertility in one of a couple

When people attend a doctor's appointment and find there is a suspected problem involving only one of the couple, both people may struggle, as this affects each differently.

It is often a shock for a man or a woman to find they have a fertility issue, and this shock and loss triggers grief. Hearing news of your compromised fertility challenges your sense of value within the couple. Letting yourself be reassured by your partner of their caring and love of you is important, as is recognising that your partner, too, will be feeling the impact of your problem. Joining to grieve together can provide a strength that will support future treatment. Recognising each other's loss and being prepared to listen carefully and accept the other's point of view is the first step to working together to cope with infertility. (Refer to 'Chapter 2: Grief—the ongoing story'.)

Things to think about

- This is a major event, so take your time to learn about it by reading, and if you have a friend or family member to confide in, do. They can be very reassuring.
- It may help to go onto the clinic website before your doctor's appointment to get some general understanding.
- Talk to your partner, and, as your sense of what is happening develops, process the changes with your partner.

- Try to have other aspects of life as part of your conversation and activities. It is easy to 'burn' your partner's ears and make them dread yet another talk that does not go anywhere different.
- Use New Zealand sources of information to become informed.

Things that may be helpful

- For most people, work is a place where we can be successful. Use this to balance the challenges you may have in getting pregnant.
- Keep all the lifestyle activities happening; they will keep you physically well and emotionally able to cope.
- Communicate with the person you feel most comfortable with in the clinic about any special needs you may have.

Chapter 8

Treatment dilemmas

Coping with acronyms

Fertility treatment is full of acronyms. They are the short way of indicating something that has a long medical term. Rather than seeking the knowledge on a website, the booklet the clinic gives you will have a glossary at the end with the abbreviation and its meaning. All of the acronyms used in the booklet will be in that glossary. (And there is a glossary at the back of this book to help with acronyms!)

It is often not necessary to understand or remember the full medical name for the acronym, but it is good to know what it means so you understand. Few people call IVF by its full name, but many understand it means 'in vitro fertilisation'.

From the time you do blood tests for your doctor's appointment you will hear acronyms. At that first appointment ask what they mean so you understand what is being talked about at the time. You can look them up later in the booklet to refresh.

Technology

Science and technology are evolving at a rapid pace in the fertility world. As the science and technology develop, the ethical issues and constraints have to develop with them. An activity that once belonged to two people, that of starting a baby, now can have many people and much technology involved. In the beginning legal, ethical and religious groups debated whether making an embryo outside of the womb was dangerous and could lead to all sorts of problems. Constraints were put around how the scientists did this, and fertility practices largely followed these ethical constraints.

Challenges still exist and fertility ethics and bioethics are evolving fields. This book wishes to acknowledge that, without delving into the field. It recognises that clinics and practitioners in New Zealand and similar countries adhere to best ethical practices.

In the early 1980s, when my partner and I were struggling with our infertility, IVF was just beginning in New Zealand. We still relied on calendars to tell us about the menstrual cycle and the first port of call was the GP. Many of the treatments used to sort out ovulation issues and blocked tubes in those days are seldom used now, as more successful treatments are available.

Science and the technologies developed, and by 2001, when I first worked at Fertility Associates, the intracytoplasmic sperm injection (ICSI)—the injecting of one sperm into an egg—was just beginning and was changing treatment for much male infertility. Prior to ICSI, a very low sperm count was treated using donor sperm, so having an option to use the man's own sperm was science at its best. Technology has moved well forward since then.

Nowadays when people arrive at the clinic they may be using an ovulation planner app on their phone to understand their menstrual cycle. They may have searched online and become informed about the problems that may occur. They come to the clinic for the doctor's expertise and diagnosis. The couple can expect to do some blood tests and the man a semen analysis prior to seeing the specialist. Generally the doctor will talk about either some further testing for one or both people, or about the appropriate treatment for their situation.

Clinics are aware that the language of fertility diagnosis and treatment can be overwhelming when people are first at the clinic. Being in a strange place with new professionals, receiving a lot of information, and the new language are all confusing and exhausting. However, it is very hard to provide the necessary information to patients without using technical language. Most patients, as they read their handbook and become more familiar with the language, become comfortable hearing the words and acronyms used. Some people ask nurses or counsellors to help them understand by explaining things in lay person's language.

Some patients need further and more sophisticated testing than the baseline testing everyone has. This requires mastering more language, thinking about whether the treatment feels appropriate, and thinking about whether it is affordable if it is not funded. It is likely the specialist will tell you about that after they have seen your initial results. Ask for information sheets and a run-down of costs so you are not trying to remember everything. It is important to know what the specialist is looking for in this testing and what the implications are if they find it.

Currently there are many diagnostic tools (and acronyms) for the testing of gametes, embryos and uterine environment. Along with this there are tools for helping make decisions about which gamete or embryo is the best to use. An example is time-lapse photography of growing embryos to help select the best to transfer. Clinics are well placed to recommend certain treatments.

Some patients either morally or financially see the tools as a step too far.

Olivia and Scott

Olivia and Scott live in a small town on an acre of land. Their home is off the grid, and their lifestyle values self-sufficiency as far as they can manage. They grow their own food, walk or bicycle to as many places as reasonable, and use as few drugs as possible in their lives. They came to the first specialist appointment and found themselves struggling with the medicalisation that was overtaking them in their quest to have a child. Fortunately they saw the nurse after the doctor and she realised they were struggling. She suggested counselling so they had a chance to talk matters through slowly and in mainly nonmedical language. This helped them to unwrap the situation and express their feelings.

Scott had a poor sperm count and they had been recommended IVF with ICSI. The doctor suggested Scott have a sperm chromatin structure assay (SCSA test) done on his sperm to look for DNA damage. It took Scott and Olivia a while to feel they understood these four acronyms.

Understanding IVF left them stunned at the drugs Olivia would have to take to make several eggs. Scott felt guilty about her needing this treatment because of his poor sperm count. They also struggled with the clinic selecting good sperm and injecting one into each egg.

The couple talked at length about how conflicting this was for them when they wanted things to be as natural as possible. They felt much better having been able to discuss it and think about alternative choices. They were eligible for a publicly funded treatment but there would be a period of waiting time before their turn came up.

The counsellor talked about other pathways they could choose, prior to undertaking IVF, which might help them both in their treatment. These would be unlikely to take away the need for treatment, but might reduce the intensity and would allow them to take some action themselves.

In the largely educational session, the counsellor told Olivia and Scott that sperm take 10 weeks from when first created in the testes to when they are mature enough to be ejaculated and fertilise an egg. She suggested the couple undertake some lifestyle changes while they waited. Scott was very enthusiastic about this, although once he knew what was being asked of him he understood it would be hard.

The doctor had suggested he take a multivitamin specific to fertility for men—a drug developed to ensure men get the right trace elements amongst other things. He could choose to minimise his alcohol intake and eliminate recreational drugs and tobacco or vaping. Scott was very still and quiet when the counsellor confirmed the importance of this, then he commented this would be difficult as not only was weed part of his daily life, it was also part of their group of friends' meetings.

The couple had a lot to consider and decisions to make about how far they were prepared to go to become parents. They did feel very supported after having a long talk about the bigger picture. Later, Scott decided to take action. This improved his sperm enough that they did not need ICSI, but they still required IVF to become pregnant. They were able to accept this.

There are an increasing number of investigations that you can be offered and you need to think about what you accept. Each of these extra investigations are likely to have an emotional and often a financial cost. It is important to talk with the doctor and ask questions about the significance of the result to the outcome, then weigh up whether it feels like a worthwhile extra.

Science and technology have created fertility opportunities that do not sit well for some cultures, beliefs and ethics. The drive to be parents means some people find their way through the conflict and others are unable to do so and have to make choices.

There are fundamental dilemmas that are a clash between what can be done and what some people believe is acceptable to be done. For some infertile people, God is asking them to accept it is His decision they do not have children. Other people challenge when life begins, and there are many different opinions on this. Some people believe it is when the sperm enters the egg, others when implantation into the uterus occurs, and still others when the embryo has a heartbeat. If someone believes that life begins with the fertilisation of an egg, or the development of an embryo, then they believe they must use them all. Discussions with the laboratory staff may provide a solution allowing the use of IVF without making too many embryos that cannot be used. These solutions can include limiting the number of eggs fertilised, or freezing excess eggs as unfertilised eggs.

Another example of the clash between technology and beliefs is the laboratory use of human albumin serum. This is against the beliefs of groups who do not like the mixing of blood products. There is an alternative, and by talking with laboratory staff you can find out about this.

Using donor gametes

When people do not have gametes that they can use successfully, they are pointed in the direction of donor gametes. This is a big consideration for people, and while many do come to terms with this, most find it a big challenge.

The use of donated eggs or sperm does not sit comfortably with some beliefs. In New Zealand all people who may use donated eggs, sperm or embryos have to have counselling. A number discuss their fear that it is tantamount to adultery in their faith. Some have talked with their church leader and become aware that their branch of the church has not had to think about this. Others are given a blanket instruction they are not to do this. Some people decide they will keep the use of donor gametes secret and just live with the guilt, such is their desire to parent. Sometimes it is helpful for couples to realise that with IVF the combining of eggs and sperm happens in the laboratory and at no time do the donated gametes go into the woman until they are part of an embryo.

Other people are aware their families would not accept them or their children if they knew they used donor gametes. This leads to the painful decision about not sharing their use of donations or remaining without children.

Sometimes people use donor embryos. These are embryos that are left over when a couple has completed their family and feel they cannot dispose of their remaining embryos. The sense of saving these embryos from storage or destruction sits comfortably with some people who struggle with donor sperm or eggs. Embryo donation is not common, as most couples cannot fathom giving away their embryos—they see this as equivalent to giving away their child.

Technology can provide another dilemma—some women using IVF create a lot of eggs. If the eggs are fertilised and most become embryos, it is likely some of the embryos won't be used. If the couple do not feel they can donate the embryos, they have the difficult decision about disposal. Clinics can store embryos for 10 years, and to keep them after that requires an ethics committee approval. The storage tanks in clinics have a great many embryos that people are finding difficult to dispose of after the effort it has taken to create them.

Respectfully disposing of embryos, eggs and sperm that cannot be used is the wish of a number of couples or individuals. There are suggestions such as putting the tubes they are stored in under a plant—a symbol of life. Occasionally a woman will get them made into a small charm for a bracelet or necklace; other people just wish to have control of their disposal. Most, however, recognise that clinics are respectful of the embryos and gametes and will dispose of them carefully.

A gentle and helpful book written by Christine Bannan and Winnie Duggan called *Be Fertile with Your Infertility* looks at ceremonies that acknowledge the importance of embryos that cannot be used.

Attempting to avoid clinic treatment and technology—natural therapies

In an effort to conceive, many people explore natural therapies to support their fertility health. Taking charge of your health and wellbeing is a good tool. This is a very personal choice for any person or couple. There are a large range of natural therapies and therapists depending on where you live. Trying out therapies that allow you to have control over what you add to your body is often a very good early undertaking, as it recognises that help is needed. It may be expensive and quite difficult to assess when to stop. Many of the natural therapies cannot be used in conjunction with clinic treatment largely because they have not been tested to discover their impact on the drugs that the clinics use. It is known that some of the herbs and medicines used in natural therapies lessen the quality of the gametes or embryos, or affect the lining of the uterus.

People need to balance their use of natural therapies with their age and the time it takes to be able to access treatment through the clinics, particularly if they wish to use publicly funded treatment. If they are paying for the clinic treatment, then the cost of both types of therapies has to be reckoned with.

Acupuncture and massage are both useful natural therapies that can run in conjunction with clinic-based treatment.

Treatment and fertility fatigue

It is easy to underestimate the toll that the lack of success and consecutive treatments take on a person or people. For some people, as the number of treatments increases or even just what is available and recommended becomes more complex, they find they have conflict between having a sense of obligation to the clinic that is looking after them and a need to step back and reflect on how much they can tolerate and afford. The need to stop and look out at life, then decide if they wish to proceed is common, and often people need support from the clinic to do this.

It is important to consider the cost both economically and emotionally and balance this with the information on success, then use this to guide yourself for what comes next.

Things to think about

- Have a look at the clinic website so you can become familiar with what to expect at the first appointment, or ask the receptionist about it on the phone.
- Do you need a support person with you? What role will this person have in the appointment—speaking or just listening?
- After the initial appointments, identify the issues.
- Read the handbook given to you, especially the sections that are important to you.
- Take time to think about it all.

Things that might be helpful

- Taking a pen, paper and questions to appointments so you are not trying to recall everything.
- Using the handbook provided, including the glossary of terms, to help you understand.
- Taking a support person in a listening role, someone you feel safe to talk with afterwards.
- Taking time to consider what is being recommended and developing a level of comfort with it.
- If donor eggs or sperm do not sit comfortably with you, talk with the counsellor about the range of options potentially available.
- If you are interested in using donor embryos, talk with your doctor and counsellor before you make up your mind—this treatment presents some extra challenges that you need to consider.

Chapter 9

Women and fertility

For many women having children in our lives is a reflection of our childhood memories and our wish to share similar activities with a child—and sometimes to do things differently. We assume we will be able to have children when we are ready.

Most women are able to conceive, carry a pregnancy and have children to parent. With 1 in 4 couples needing fertility support, there are a portion of heterosexual women who need fertility treatment to make this possible. In addition, women in same-gender relationships, or who are trans, or single and wish to parent by themselves, are likely to use fertility treatment.

Regardless of the reason they need the treatment, most women find the process challenging. Accepting the medical profession into our reproductive lives and following the requirements of the treatment programmes have a cost to us. The drugs, the scans, and the gamete or embryo placement into the uterus all have some impact on us. When successful, we are able to put this aside and focus on the outcome. When there is a lack of success or a need for ongoing treatment, the cost, emotional and economic, may be high and our sense of self impacted.

It is easy for fertility treatment to dominate our lives. Seeing treatment as one part of life and ensuring we keep the other parts of our life whole and proceeding normally is helpful. By maintaining the other aspects of life, such as friendships, family support, being effective at work and talking with our partner or a close friend, we get through this phase of life.

Understanding the impact of upbringing

Women's roles in our society have changed, as a result of feminism and women being successful in careers and as income-earners. Many of us have careers and paid work while continuing to be the primary carer in the home.

Women and men have embedded attitudes and beliefs picked up from childhood, from their culture and from popular TV shows that show women as primarily the nurturers with responsibility for raising children within a family. Children may see their mother doing most of the parenting alongside having a career.

Parents can provide neutral role models, but the way they fulfill life's tasks and the ways they interact with others creates strong impressions on their children. Little girls grow up to see women become mothers, to see pregnancy, and then the joy of those around them with the new baby. This suggests that becoming a parent is attractive and gets a lot of positive feedback, and so they too may wish to do this.

Parents communicate their expectations of and to their daughters from an early age. They teach little girls to communicate more gently and use discussion as a tool, and they are happy to foster activities such as dance and creativity. Girls often role-play, including some playing being mother. The socialisation of female children includes a level of focus on their future role as mothers. At puberty girls learn about the purpose of menstrual cycles, and begin to become aware of the purpose of their body producing eggs. This knowledge coincides with their body maturing and becoming prepared for pregnancy.

It seems as if as soon as fertility is mentioned it engages many women. In early adulthood women are likely to have a level of focus on menstrual cycles and preventing pregnancy. Most girls enjoy chatting with their friends, and they will discuss their physical development and its meaning as well as changing attractions and relationships with their friends. They get their information from friends, family, the internet and literature geared towards their age group. Fertility, both controlling it and accessing it, is synonymous with women. Most women have an interest in everything to do with fertility, contraception, pregnancy and birth, and raising children. They spend time reading, talking and thinking about this topic. This interest develops as their family and friends have children and wish to share aspects of the experience.

Adolescent girls may care for younger siblings and other children and earn pocket money through babysitting. At the appropriate time they learn to deal with periods, their changing bodies, contraception and relationships. As they mature and think forward, having children comes into focus and they think about the role parenting may have in their future. In their choice of career many young women consider the impact of stopping work to have a child and how that will affect their career expectations. They sometimes choose careers that can accommodate this.

Preparing to be a parent

In New Zealand, a woman's average age at the birth of her first child is 31. Many women wish to work before they start to have children. This may be to progress their career or to pay off student loans and maybe purchase their first home. Our expectation is that we will be able to become pregnant when we wish. We have an internal voice that reminds us as we reach our thirties that fertility has a timeline that must be considered. When a pregnancy does not occur we become concerned. This is the fear of not being able to become a parent. At the time when friends are having children, women look towards belonging to the community of mothers. When we are not successful, it may lead to a sense of loss of womanhood and a questioning of how we fit into the community. Fortunately, a number of us act upon this anxiety by seeking information and investigating.

Women and lifestyle

Conception and pregnancy are advantaged when we take time to plan how we will integrate the lifestyle issues that may benefit us and the hoped-for child. Having a healthy body and lifestyle, and taking supplements such as folic acid, promote these aspects.

This preparation works in favour of conception and a healthy pregnancy and child, whether using fertility help or succeeding naturally. Some of the things to consider are as follows.

Folic acid

All women hoping to become pregnant should take a folic-acid supplement. Very early in pregnancy the spinal cord begins development, and the chance of neural tube defects is increased when there is insufficient folic acid. An example of what can happen is spina bifida, where the neural tube that surrounds and protects the spinal cord does not develop sufficiently and can result in paralysis from the waist down. This happens very early in pregnancy, so often a woman may not realise she is pregnant when this occurs. Taking folic acid prior to conception will prevent this. There are a number of other reasons to take folic acid; your specialist will discuss this with you.

Smoking and vaping

The New Zealand Ministry of Health states that the woman must have been a non-smoker or non-vaper for at least three months before being successfully scored for publicly funded treatment. Nicotine can pass the placental barrier and negatively impact on a foetus and its cardiorespiratory development. Babies of mothers who smoked during pregnancy have lower birth weights, are more likely to need time in a neonatal unit, and are at increased risk of sudden infant death syndrome. Nicotine can also be passed to baby through breast milk, and this is thought to disrupt babies' sleep patterns, make babies more susceptible to sudden infant death syndrome, and influence the development of allergy-related illness, such as asthma, in children.

Alcohol

Alcohol is not safe to drink while trying to become pregnant, during pregnancy or while breastfeeding. Babies can develop foetal alcohol syndrome, which creates lifelong learning and behavioural disorders. As the brain of a foetus develops right through pregnancy, drinking alcohol at any stage can have an impact on the child.

Weight

As with all aspects of health, having a lifestyle that ensures women are a healthy body mass index (BMI) of 20–25 is significant in helping fertility. Women who are either underweight or overweight are likely to have difficulties conceiving and are harder to treat successfully and safely. The Ministry of Health funding is quite specific about a woman having a BMI of under 32. This acknowledges that as a woman has more fatty tissue she is less likely to ovulate, and the quantity of drugs needed to help her provide eggs is higher, and the drugs are generally less successful. In addition, the risk of developing conditions such as diabetes and high blood pressure in pregnancy is higher when women are carrying more weight.

Women who have a BMI of 18 and under are also harder to treat and have a greater risk in pregnancy.

Exercise

Maintaining a good level of fitness is beneficial for the woman's body and her mind. Understanding what amount of exercise is required for a woman to feel fit is different for each individual. Too much exercise can impact on ovulation; however, some exercise can really support a woman's body in the quest to become pregnant. Targeting moderate exercise will give the benefits of exercise, help with controlling weight, and maintain the psychological benefits that exercise brings.

Caffeine

As part of fertility treatment women are encouraged to reduce, and if possible eliminate, caffeine from their diet. Caffeine is found in coffee, tea, energy drinks and fizzy drinks such as Coke, Pepsi and Mountain Dew, with lower levels found in chocolate and cocoa. While trying to become pregnant and during pregnancy, keeping caffeine consumption low is recommended.

Food and drink

Eating a well-balanced diet with plenty of vegetables and fruit is good for all people and ensures that pregnant and breastfeeding women will be able to nourish their child. Dietitians use a food pyramid to indicate the amounts of each food type so the diet is balanced. There are some trace elements that are low in New Zealand soils, and therefore in our foods, which are important as they advantage the development of the foetus. Both folic acid and iodine are in this category. Many doctors recommend iodine to enhance baby's brain development.

Water and low-fat milk are the most recommended drinks for women who are trying to become pregnant. Women can also have caffeine-free herbal teas, small amounts of fruit juice (juice is high in sugar) and some soft drinks in moderation. It is important to maintain a good level of hydration, and water is the best drink to do this.

Chemicals that may affect fertility

Recent studies are showing that a particular group of chemicals called endocrine disrupting chemicals (EDCs) may have negative effects on both women and men's reproductive capacity.

EDCs occur naturally in some foods, soil and water, but not in sufficient amounts to impact on us. However, some plastics, personal-care items and food wrappings contain higher levels of these chemicals. While it is not known how exactly individual chemicals affect our health, studies have shown that EDCs mimic or block oestrogen and testosterone. By changing our hormone levels they can impact on egg and sperm numbers, change the DNA, and affect the capacity to achieve and hold a pregnancy.

A few simple ways of reducing the amount we absorb include washing all fruit and vegetables before eating, buying as few pre-packaged products as possible, and being careful in your use of plastic water bottles and food containers, especially when heating food.

Women and age

Women are at the peak of their fertility in their mid-to late twenties. There is a slow decline in the number of eggs and the genetic material in the eggs up to about 36 years. This decline speeds up in the later thirties and early forties, and by the mid-forties a woman will find it difficult to become pregnant using her own eggs.

If a woman in her late thirties or early forties needs treatment and wishes to have more than one child, she will need to raise this with the specialist so her treatment maximises her chance of having more than one child. An example of this occurs when a woman has IVF and her ovaries are stimulated to produce a number of eggs. If she ends up with several embryos and has a child with the first or second, she can use the remaining embryos for another child. Embryos do not age when frozen, so she may well have a good chance of more than one child.

Megan

Megan was 41 when she came to the clinic to talk with both the doctor and the counsellor. She had suddenly become aware of the implications of her age and recognised having a child might not be straightforward. She had a successful and satisfying career in the media world and felt ready to have children. She did not have a partner but did have a single friend who was willing to be the sperm donor. He was not a parent either and they discussed the idea of being co-parents. They saw that as the best option for all three of them. Megan began reading about fertility and pregnancy and felt significant anxiety that she had left it this long. She began the lifestyle changes she felt would benefit a pregnancy.

Megan wanted everything to happen quickly. She accepted IVF would be her best option and wanted all her tests and those of her donor to be completed quickly so she could just begin the treatment. She was aware of and comfortable with the costs of treatment.

The testing of Megan's fertility brought her unwelcome news. Her tests showed a diminished fertility as the age statistics had suggested was likely. She just wanted to get going with her treatment.

Megan's frustration rose with the process of the donation and the quarantining the sperm had to undergo. She felt she knew enough about her donor that she should be able to voluntarily forgo this. She understood clinics needed to have protocols but found them inconvenient.

Eventually Megan and her friend had IVF and made three embryos. Their first embryo did not create a pregnancy and it was with trepidation she had the second embryo replaced. She became pregnant and sadly miscarried at six weeks. On her third try Megan was truly anxious. She now knew that getting pregnant was the first step and staying pregnant the second. She worked hard to manage her anxiety and used alternative therapies such as acupuncture and yoga to help her. Luckily she was rewarded with an ongoing pregnancy and in due course a healthy daughter.

Megan was keen to share her story as she realised how lucky she was at now 42 to have a child. She wanted to alert others to begin the process earlier.

Women, careers and children

Society values education and recognises it provides a means to having a job and lifestyle, including the security of a home and the capacity to provide well for children. While not everybody has the opportunity to access education, many do undertake tertiary education and often use a student loan to facilitate this.

At the conclusion of tertiary education women may feel the need to consolidate a career and pay off some student loan debt; hence the average age of 31 before having their first child.

Some women are older when they meet their partner, take time to live within the relationship and then feel ready to embark on having a family.

Women may wish to extend their options by undertaking egg freezing while they are younger and still producing reasonable numbers of eggs that are likely to be good quality. Approaching a fertility clinic and having the opportunity to discuss this and do some basic testing to see if this is an option is a good strategy.

A portion of women desire to have a career and to be recognised as highly competent and receive promotions or move up the career pathway by transferring to other firms for advancement. These aspirations may come at a cost. Women in senior positions may be older and find it harder to become pregnant and then to take parental leave and juggle the needs of small children. Having children often means women need to work differently at this phase of life. Some male partners are prepared to be primary caregivers for their young child or to share the responsibility with the mother to enable her to continue in her work.

Other women, either partnered or single, wish to have both a career that is satisfying and children as part of their life plan, but they do not necessarily aspire towards the glass ceiling in their work. They act within the fertile years of their lives. This may mean planning well in advance, particularly if the woman is planning to use donor sperm. Getting onto the list for the use of donor sperm for both single women and those in same-gender relationships is important since the wait can be more than 18 months.

Planning parental leave is necessary for many women. In New Zealand they can have 26 weeks of paid parental leave, after which they need a strategy for coping economically or for childcare for their young child. Working and being the primary parent for a young child is a big task for anyone.

Women and the media

Women's magazines, TV shows and 'chick lit' all influence women's perceptions of themselves and their options in life. Stories are a powerful medium to provide information and suggest ways women can run their lives. Stories of course are not always the whole truth and may imply less-than-useful information. An example of this is the female stars of film and TV who have children in their late forties. Statistically it is very unlikely they have used their own eggs to conceive, even with the best technology available. But they do not talk about this in the articles. It is implied they conceived with medical intervention such as IVF. This will be true but only part of the truth—the IVF may have happened to include an egg donor and they had an embryo replaced.

Being careful about accepting the stories where the information seems unusual is a good strategy. It will be impossible to know whether any story is actually correct but it's important to understand the impacts of increased egg age—their diminished number with increasing age, the DNA in the nucleus becoming less viable, the embryo's reduced capacity to implant, and increases in miscarriage. Statistically a woman's chance of using her own eggs and producing a live birth at 45 is under 2 per cent.

Things to think about

- Do you see children as being part of your future?
- Have you considered the effects of aging and how that can be integrated into the plan for the next part of your life?
- How would it be if there were no children?
- What investigations might you do to ensure you have options to wait a while before you embark on baby-making?
- How can you as a woman protect your fertility and your future options?

Things that might be helpful

- Information is a powerful tool in making decisions. Some of this will be general information about fertility and the future. Other information may be about your specific chances—this can be obtained to a large part through blood tests.

- Making plans for the future and having children as part of these plans. Timing can be incorporated into these plans.
- Being aware of the financial support available from the government and of your employers' attitudes to parental leave.
- Being aware of the activities that support self-esteem, and maintaining them.

Chapter 10

Men and fertility

Men, like women, come in all shapes and sizes, and with a variety of levels of knowledge about their bodies and also of their partner's reproductive system. Most of the time this is not an issue, but when there is trouble conceiving it may place men on the back foot. This, combined with the sense that conception, pregnancy and having a child involve women more than men, may make some men feel excluded.

Fertility investigations and the drive for treatment are generally initiated by women. Men are generally supportive partners, but for many the investigations and treatment are bewildering.

Sometimes the news from the fertility specialist tells the man that his body is part or all of the issue. He may not have suspected issues as he is able to make love and ejaculate perfectly normally, and since semen makes the majority of the ejaculate it is unlikely he will notice a problem.

Men can have issues with the numbers of sperm, the morphology (shape and size), with DNA damage done in the 10-week passage through the testes, or with an absence of sperm from an injury, genetic condition or childhood issue. In addition there are times when lifestyle factors may have an impact on the number and quality of the sperm. In some instances the specialist is able to help with the production of sperm and will talk with the man about this. In other instances there may be nothing that can be done, and the couple may have to consider donor sperm.

Nick

Nick will never forget the sense of falling into a deep hole when the doctor told him he had no sperm. A scramble of thoughts leapt into his head. Who was he if he did not have the capacity to create a child? Why in this scientific era could they not fix this problem? Would Kathy still love him? Did his family need to know? As the only son so much depended on him having a son to carry on the family story. What was his worth now?

Nick, like many men, associated his ability to produce sperm with his manliness and felt he was less of a man as a result of having no sperm. He talked of his fear that his family and friends would see him as a less worthy man. Indeed he feared teasing from his friends if he told them.

Fortunately Nick had his partner Kathy with him at the appointment, and while he simply went blank and wanted out of the doctor's office, Kathy was able to listen and have her questions answered. She asked if there was a possibility of seeing the counsellor so they could get some support before leaving, and the doctor talked with the counsellor who was able to give them a short crisis appointment before they left the clinic.

At counselling Nick and Kathy's greatest need was to sort out how to manage the next few days so they could get over the shock of this news and make a plan of how to proceed. Kathy wept in counselling because she was unsure how to support her man. Nick was able to comfort her, and at that first counselling session she affirmed for him that he was her love and she had married him for the person he was and not for the babies they might make together.

Nick felt able to talk in counselling because he trusted the confidentiality and he did not have to see the counsellor any other time in his life except when he initiated it. Over time Nick and Kathy used counselling to come to terms with their issue. Nick went separately a couple of times as he worked through his guilt at not being able to produce sperm and of Kathy needing treatment because of him. Nick had to work hard to assimilate the information about his lack of sperm and integrate this into his sense of himself. He had to work to overcome the sense of guilt and shame he had originally associated with infertility in men. As his acceptance of himself and the situation increased, he regained his desire for intimacy with Kathy and was eventually able to weigh up the question: 'How much do we want to be parents?'

Nick and Kathy talked, over quite a long time, about how they would resolve the lack of sperm, as they had decided they wished to parent. Nick did not want Kathy to miss out on the experience of carrying and birthing children. Nick was the last male in his immediate family and he knew the genes were important to his family, who were very proud of their heritage. He eventually summoned the courage to ask his first cousin to donate sperm, and the cousin agreed to do this. They decided to tell his immediate family once Kathy was pregnant. When they did tell them, the family's first reaction was shock but they were then glad to welcome their grandchild.

Issues for men

While the cause of lack of sperm for Nick was unknown, there are several reasons men may have troubles with their sperm.

A relatively small number of men have undescended testes at birth and, depending on what happens following birth, they may or may not be able to produce sperm. A generation ago parents were told that as long as they dropped the testes before puberty all should be well. Now it is known the sooner the testes are dropped into the scrotum the better for the chances of having sperm.

Genetic conditions specific to men such as Klinefelter syndrome may cause the loss of production of sperm. Klinefelter syndrome is a relatively random chromosomal disorder that occurs when a male is born with an additional X chromosome. While this genetic condition has a number of likely symptoms, lack of sperm production seems to affect most men with it.

Other genetic conditions can also affect sperm production or quality. In the case of a man who has cystic fibrosis he may not have a vas deferens. The sperm may exist in the testes but not be able to be released. Surgical sperm retrieval will be available to this couple, producing immature but usable sperm. As well as obtaining sperm this way there will be testing of his partner to ensure she is not a cystic fibrosis carrier. If she is found to be a carrier the couple will need to have their embryos tested so their children do not have cystic fibrosis. They will be offered PGD, preimplantation genetic diagnosis. Prior to that the couple will have genetic counselling to fully understand the condition and chances of affecting a subsequent child. If they require PGD then the embryos will be tested, with only the unaffected or carrier embryos being available for use. If the woman is not a carrier they will move to the next step. IVF will follow and any embryos will be grown and used.

At other times male infertility is only diagnosed after a period of lack of success at treatment. The specialist will have requested a further blood test called a karyotype, which may provide this information. This may reveal a variation from the normal chromosome number, and the specialist will recommend what happens following this diagnosis.

A further issue that may affect some men is erectile issues. There can be many reasons for this, and often there is a need for hormonal and chromosomal testing to try to identify the cause. This may require medical or psychological support.

Impact of fertility issues on a man

Regardless of the reason for the male issues with infertility, it is a huge blow and significant grief for a man to hear that he has fertility issues. It may take days of grappling with the feelings of sadness and often frustration or anger for the man to be ready to talk about it and to accept his partner's support.

If the man has coupled his fertility and ability to produce children with his sense of manliness, it will take time, reflection and support for the man to regain his balance. He is, effectively, the person he was before he got that news, but inside him there may be doubt about himself and the need to think through and learn to recognise that not everything has changed about him; the many things he is good at still remain. He will need to accept himself.

There are a number of things that impact on him—the loss of privacy as testing is done, the fear about others' reactions if he shares the information, the psychological assumptions about parenthood that may need to be rewritten. The impact on his self-confidence needs to be recognised. His feelings about himself in his relationship and the impact this has on his partner are all part of coming to terms with this. This does not happen quickly, and the couple may have similar conversations a number of times until the man is able to accept the new version of himself.

Specific to men is the situation where his woman may be fertile and may need fertility treatment because of his condition. Fertility treatment in most cases largely happens to women, as the eggs will need to be collected so the sperm can be coupled with or injected into them. This requires stimulation with injections to get several eggs and then an egg collection. Men can support their partner well through this process by accepting they are in this treatment together. Watching the person he loves undertake this treatment can create a sense of guilt. Men need to be aware that their partner would probably prefer to undergo treatment so they have the opportunity of their having a child together.

Ashley and Andy

Ashley and Andy were parenting her child from her previous relationship and decided to grow their family. When no pregnancy occurred they sought help and discovered Andy had low sperm numbers. The doctor told them they would need ICSI, the intracytoplasmic sperm injection (where one sperm is placed inside each egg) to have a child together.

He then explained the process of IVF and gave them some reading.

Andy hated the thought of IVF for Ashley and could not understand how accepting she was of the need for it. He finally allowed himself to hear how much she wanted to have a child with him and recognise her happiness that they had a chance at having a child together.

Relationships are about sharing both joys and troubles. It is allowing the person you love to support and comfort you when there is something to accept. It is helpful to both people to work together to cope with the situation.

Treatment for men

Most fertility treatment happens to women, but a woman cannot have treatment without having sperm to help create an embryo. The process of producing a sperm sample may be challenging, especially in the clinic. Clinics need relatively fresh samples and so if you are travelling a distance you may need to produce it at the clinic. If you fail to produce a sample when it is needed, the doctor may suggest drugs or other means of getting your sperm.

Sometimes men do not have sperm in their ejaculate but hormone tests indicate they may have sperm in their testes. For these men a surgical sperm retrieval can be performed. When this happens the specialist does a fine-needle biopsy of the testes, with pain relief, to extract immature sperm that can then be frozen, ready to be injected into the eggs. If sperm is collected this way the laboratory will freeze it so it can be used in successive treatments if needed. Men will need to have a quiet few days following this procedure, as the swelling reduces and healing happens.

Sometimes there is no possibility of sperm and the couple will be faced with a decision: to parent, they will need to use donor sperm. This is a big step and requires that the couple consider what is important to them. Is it the genetic connection or is it the raising of children? Being a good parent is not dependent on a genetic connection, it is about the quality of time and energy you put into parenting.

Donor sperm can come from a personal donor—someone you know and trust. This may give you the opportunity to have some of your genes in your children if you have a suitable brother or cousin. Sometimes a friend is the best option. For some people there is no suitable personal donor option so investigating whether the clinic donors will work for you is a good move. Talking to the counsellor, who has a lot of experience in donors and donations, getting onto the waiting lists and then letting time go by is a strategy here. As the wait nears the end, take some time to talk and think about what you might realistically want in a donor.

Using donor sperm is not for everyone and some couples decide they will explore other options, such as adoption, fostering or being child-free.

Lifestyle influences for men

As with women there are a number of lifestyle factors that have a direct influence on the fertility of men. Keep in mind: sperm takes about 10 weeks from production to being mature enough to fertilise an egg. These lifestyle factors can impact on sperm at any stage, so being proactive in correcting them will take time to show the benefit.

Tobacco and recreational drugs

Smoking, vaping and recreational drugs can all affect sperm quality and should be avoided when trying to conceive.

Alcohol

Some alcohol will be unlikely to affect sperm production and quality, but keeping alcohol consumption to 15 units a week or under is recommended.

Diet

Eating healthy food and a good variety of fruit and vegetables should provide the right minerals and trace elements. When there is some doubt that the diet is sufficient, the man should explore taking a fertility supplement to support his sperm production. While caffeine does not have a direct impact on sperm, moderation of caffeine and an increase in drinking water are beneficial to all people.

Normal BMI

Keeping weight within the normal BMI (18.5–24.9) helps fertility. Overweight men most often have a sedentary lifestyle. Sitting with a large tummy and legs surrounding the testes may overheat them, and overheating sperm can cause them to die in the testes. Exercise is helpful both to control the weight and to give stronger abdominal muscles to support the tummy above the testes.

It is generally recommended that men who have low sperm numbers or quality wear boxer shorts rather than underpants under trousers, to provide air circulation around the testes and keep them cool.

Chemicals that impact on fertility

As stated in 'Chapter 9: Women and fertility', recent studies are showing that a particular group of chemicals called endocrine disrupting chemicals (EDCs) may have negative effects on both women and men's reproductive capacity. (See section entitled "Chemicals that may affect fertility" for more detail.)

Things to think about

- You may find yourself asking questions such as 'Am I still the same person as I was yesterday, before I found out?' or 'Will my partner continue to love me?' This is natural.
- Do other people need to know what's going on, or can you keep it quiet?
- Are you worried that if you tell friends they will say inappropriate things about not being a real man? Are there people you can trust?
- Grief is really personal but can have a huge impact on the people around you. How will you know if others

such as your partner are not coping with the infertility?

- What will you do to keep your world going?

Things that may be helpful

- Being together at the specialist appointment, and recognising that you will be likely to pick up different things in the conversation.
- Asking for written information if the clinic has some, so you can read it and digest at a later time.
- Seeking someone to talk with—this may be the counsellor or the doctor's nurse.
- Taking time to talk as a couple, but taking care to not let this be the only topic of conversation.
- Remembering who you were before this news and ensuring you retain the friendships and activities of that life.
- Exploring the options to parenthood suggested by the specialist.
- Thinking about your father and his fathering of you. What do you remember with pleasure about your relationship with him? Are these

things because of the genetic link or because, as a dad, he interacted well with you?

- If a donor is the way to parent, finding out the advantages and disadvantages of a personal donor versus a clinic donor.

Chapter 11

Same-gender relationships

Same-gender or gay relationships, like all other relationships, are about love and wanting a life with your partner of choice. Finding the right person to love and accepting their love are gifts to be cherished.

With the Human Rights Act 1993 specifically forbidding discrimination based on sexual preference, society is moving to being more inclusive. While there are still some areas that are challenging for gay couples, surrogacy and adoption now have a similar process for gay and heterosexual couples. While most of the availability to fertility treatment is the same as for heterosexual people, one difference is access to public funding, which is harder for gay relationships. This happens because in heterosexual couples both people may have fertility problems that add to the points scored, but this does not happen with gay relationships.

Same-gender couples, single women, trans people and single men are regarded as having social infertility, which means a donor is needed to provide either eggs or sperm to form an embryo. Sometimes one person may have medical infertility as well, and occasionally this can mean they qualify for funded treatment.

Same-gender female couples use the clinics to seek safe treatment with the capacity for their children to eventually meet their donor. Male couples need both an egg donor and surrogacy (see 'Chapter 15: Surrogacy'). When this is done through home insemination, the surrogate is also the egg donor; through a clinic they can have two different people in these roles.

New Zealand, along with Australia and the United Kingdom, has strong regulatory frameworks for the clinics to work within. Prior to 2004, in New Zealand, the use of donor treatment for women involved either coming to the clinic to use a clinic donor or using home insemination (finding a male donor and inseminating outside of the clinic). The clinic donors were able at this time to elect to be anonymous, although clinics encouraged them to consider the wellbeing of the children born as a result of the donation and only a relatively small portion made the choice to be anonymous. Using a home insemination required some contact between the woman and the donor, but often they chose to stay relatively unidentifiable.

In 2004 the Human Assisted Reproductive Technology (HART) Act came into law. For same-gender relationships the main area of concern was section 3 on donations. It specifies that a child or young person has a right to their genetic information, and advises clinics to collect and hold certain non-identifying information, which is available to the guardian of the donor child or young person before they are 18. At 18, or earlier in some circumstances, the young person has the right to their genetic information. In some instances the guardians can ask for the identifying information from the clinics. This means all donors have to be prepared to be available to the young people at 18 because the fertility clinics or Births, Deaths and Marriages (part of the Department of Internal Affairs) must give the young people this identity information on request. Many of the donors indicate in their profiles that they are willing to be approached about further information or contact earlier than 18.

For personal donors there is generally an agreement between the parents and the donor about how they will inform the child and the donor's other children, if any. This agreement means the child is likely to know of the donation and identity of the donor from an earlier age. The clinics must still comply with keeping the information for these young people, even if they are unlikely to need it.

In New Zealand when a same-gender female couple register a child at birth they use their names as the parents who birthed the child. These names are used for the birth certificate and they will be the legal and liable parents for the wellbeing of the young people for life. There is no option to name the donor, and indeed when donors donate they seldom want to be named or have a parenting role to the child.

It was in 2013 with the Marriage Amendment Act that joint adoption (adoption by both people) became possible for married same-sex couples. Following a High Court ruling in December 2015, any couple, married or not, became able to adopt children. With the 2013 law change, treatment became available to male couples through the fertility clinic. Men require a surrogate to have a child, and surrogacy currently requires the capacity to adopt the child after birth. Gay men were not able to do that until the Marriage Amendment Act entered into force.

Currently, when surrogacy is used by a same-gender male couple, the child will be registered by the surrogate who, with her partner, is a birth parent. The men have limited guardianship for medical issues only at birth; they will have full guardianship when the interim adoption order is signed, and when the adoption is finalised a new birth certificate is written with them as the parents.

Same-gender female couples

'Chapter 12: Using a donor—eggs and sperm' holds much of the information needed on using a donor. While women in this situation understand they will need donor sperm to make a child, there are variations in their intentions. In some instances one partner will wish to carry the child(ren) for the couple, and in other couples both women hope to carry a child and to use the same donor so the children are half siblings. Regardless of who carries the child in pregnancy, both women are full and liable parents to any child born within their relationship.

Finding a donor takes care and thought. Some women ask a friend or have another personal donor; other women do not have anyone they can ask to be their donor and will need a clinic donor.

Finding a donor

Personally recruited donors

There are advantages to using a personally recruited donor. These include the couple knowing about the man and being able to ask questions directly to him as they parent. The mothers are likely to be asked by their child, at about three years old, why some children have a daddy and they don't. The answer to this is they have two mothers and a donor who helped them create the child. They will probably not be asked at this point who the donor is, but when this occurs, and in agreement with the donor's wishes about identifiability, they can tell the child about their friend. This provides the child with knowledge of their genetic origins and helps with formation of the child's identity. A further advantage is that the treatment can happen more quickly, without the long waiting entailed with the donor waiting list.

Charlotte and Kat

Charlotte and Kat came to the clinic to discuss donor sperm. They were unsure about using a stranger as the genetic parent for their child. They were clear their child would need to know of donor and considered the best answer to 'Who is my donor?' was 'He's a friend of ours.'

Kat had someone in mind—the partner of her friend. She had mentioned to the friend that they would need a donor, and the friend had asked if they had considered her partner. Kat had said that she and Charlotte would talk about this before they went further. They had obviously talked a lot and got stuck, so came to counselling. The issues these women raised included:

• How do we ask him—through his partner or directly?

• What is the process he will have to go through?

• These people are good friends. What will it be like to have our children being half-siblings with their children?

- What if the children look very alike?
- What if other people notice the similarity?
- When would we tell the children of their relationship?
- Our families are likely to ask who the donor is. Do we tell them the truth or something else, and what is that to be?
- What is other people's experience of this?

Charlotte and Kat had an in-depth discussion about these issues and decided that since the friend had raised using her partner, Kat would go back to her friend and ask if she had spoken to her partner about the donation. The two couples would then be able to talk further.

Charlotte and Kat went around to talk with the couple, and recommended they come to counselling to consider all the implications before they agreed. They then all came to a joint counselling session where, with the safety and guidance of the counsellor, they discussed the implications of the donation for all parties, including current and potential children.

Charlotte had IVF treatment and conceived, and she and Kat are now the parents of a toddler. They have embryos in the freezer if they decide to have another child.

One hard aspect of wanting to use a personal donor is asking the man if he will donate. This can feel as though you are putting the friendship on the line. It requires courage and the ability to recognise that while he is likely to be flattered by the request, he or his partner may say no. If he agrees, then there will need to be discussion about how to manage relationships in the future and when they are likely to inform the children on both sides about their genetic connection as half-siblings. They will also need to talk about who they can tell about the donation.

Clinic-recruited donors

Clinic donors are available for both IUI (intrauterine insemination) and IVF. The clinic manages these lists on a basis that when the woman reaches the top of the list, she will be offered the choice of available donors. There is generally a significant wait for a donor.

Gemma and Holly

Gemma and Holly arrived from the United Kingdom to settle in New Zealand and did not have the networks to find a personal donor. They explored the web looking for a donor, but were warned off using a web-sourced stranger and home inseminations by other women couples. This left them a clinic donor as an option.

They were both still in their twenties and both wanted to carry a child, with Holly wanting to be first. A blood test, AMH, found Holly had good ovarian reserve, and they decided with the specialist that they would get her tubes tested to ensure they were clear, and all going well they would proceed to IUI. The nearly two-year wait (that existed at the time they were in the clinic) was longer than they had hoped for, but being practical women they decided to use the time to save some more funds, have a visit to their families and work on their home.

While some people are attracted to the anonymity of the clinic and an unknown donor, they need to consider how they will manage when the child is curious about their donor and the donor has stated they do not want contact until the young person is 18. Girls especially, often at puberty, become curious about their genetic origins. 'Chapter 13: Donor sperm' is relevant here.

Treatments for same-gender female couples

Treatment can take place either through IUI, intrauterine insemination, or through IVF, in vitro fertilisation. There are a number of factors that will dictate the appropriateness of one or the other treatment. The choice of treatment type will be made in conjunction with the fertility specialist who will look at the results of a number of tests and make a recommendation.

IUI takes place when a woman's cycle is monitored and ovulation is identified. The sperm is defrosted and placed into her uterus at the appropriate cycle time, and a pregnancy test done two weeks later. These cycles can be done in a woman's natural cycle or the cycle can be manufactured. The doctor, in discussion with the couple, will assess the woman and recommend a treatment pathway. Use of IUI will depend on a number of factors, including the woman's egg reserve, the presence of conditions such as endometriosis or polycystic ovaries, tubal function, age, and likelihood of success.

IVF, in vitro fertilisation, may be the recommended option for treatment. During IVF the woman takes fertility drugs to prepare a number of eggs, and these will be collected and fertilised by the donor sperm in the laboratory. The embryos created will be grown for five days to the blastocyst stage, the best one replaced into her uterus, and any other viable embryos frozen. IVF may be the advised treatment by the specialist if the ovarian reserve is low, or if there is endometriosis, polycystic ovaries or blocked tubes. It is sometimes the treatment of choice because of age or one person wanting to provide the eggs and the other carry the child. IVF may also be the only option if a personal donor has sperm only suitable for IVF.

Before a couple or person makes the decision about treatment they need to look into the process of the treatments, the costs involved, the potential success rates and, if they use IVF, how they would feel if they had embryos they were not going to use. Some female couples arrive at the clinic thinking they may have a child with each person's genes and the same donor. If the first woman has IVF, has a child and has frozen embryos, it becomes a huge decision to use the second woman's eggs and ultimately discard the unwanted embryos.

Same-gender male couples

For men, the capacity to adopt has allowed clinics to assist them to become parents. This book will only deal with clinic-assisted surrogacy. The men require either an egg donor or an embryo donor, or they can use donor eggs with donor sperm, and they need a surrogate to be able to carry the child. While clinics may have egg donors who are happy to donate to men, many men have the capacity to find an egg donor within their own network. Embryo donors equally can be clinic-recruited or personally recruited; donor sperm plus donor egg can be a combination of clinic-and personally recruited. Finding a surrogate is more often an issue. Clinics are not allowed to connect surrogates and intending parents, and advertising for a surrogate is illegal under the HART Act 2004.

There are a number of ways men find surrogates. This might be through their friends and family, or some ask their Facebook friends if they know anyone who wishes to be a surrogate, while others go onto surrogacy

(New-Zealand based) websites and look there. When the men find someone to be a surrogate they need to form a strong relationship with her and her family. Having someone carry your child involves trust from both sides. The men need to trust that the woman will look after herself and the child she carries and will give them the child following birth. The woman needs to feel confident the men will support her during the pregnancy, take the child following birth and be good parents. Surrogacy is a long process—ethical approval, an egg-donor cycle, pregnancy and at least three months' recovery for the woman following pregnancy. It may take two years to get through all of this, and both parties will consider this in the counselling for applying for ethical approval.

Men often come to the clinic to discuss and become familiar with the process as they begin to explore what they need to do and how to approach the various stages. Currently in New Zealand they need to begin by seeking approval for IVF Surrogacy Adoption from Oranga Tamariki. This approval is different and generally briefer than the approval for adopting a child from a stranger. However it is not a fast process.

Entering the world of fertility is opening a door to a lot of information gay men have not needed in the past. They may not know a lot about a woman's menstrual cycle, but this information, plus knowing what makes a good egg donor and about the IVF she will undergo, will help them find an egg donor and understand what they are asking her to undertake. The counsellor is probably the person who has the most time available to have a robust discussion about these facts.

Information about surrogacy and pregnancy is not always easily available to male couples. Women tend to have conversations about pregnancy and birth as they have children or watch their friends go through this. Male couples need to seek out information about the physical impact of pregnancy, the development of a child and the emotional effect on the birth mother. Some male couples, when alerted to this, are able to seek this information through their family and friends. Others may need to seek it at the clinic. Attending courses such as antenatal courses towards the end of pregnancy provides a lot of information.

Ethical approval

For gay men to begin the ethical process they need to have found a suitable surrogate. All cases of surrogacy must have case-by-case approval from the ethics committee ECART (Ethics Committee on Assisted Reproductive Technology). The process for this ensures, as far as possible, the safety of all parties and their families. Through the medical, counselling and legal interviews the participants will become informed about the implications and risks of surrogacy. They will become aware of any situations that the clinic and/or ECART regard as a risk that makes proceeding inappropriate.

Further information about ethical approval for surrogacy can be found in 'Chapter 15: Surrogacy'.

Steve and Paul

Steve and Paul came to the clinic to learn about surrogacy; they wanted to do it in the way that took best care of all parties. They had a close friend keen to be an egg donor, and after talking to their network a friend of a friend had offered to be the surrogate. They had only met this woman, Jamie, once, and they felt they might like her.

The men learned about next steps—getting in touch with Oranga Tamariki for IVF Surrogacy Adoption approval and getting to know the surrogate and her family, and beginning to formulate with her an idea of how the pregnancy and birth might proceed. They became aware of the process for ethical approval and the timeframe for the whole process.

Steve and Paul reappeared in counselling about three months later. They had seen the fertility specialist and had decided they would fertilise half of the eggs each. Neither man had issues with their sperm or their health.

Over a period of about five months the men, their surrogate and their egg donor completed their medical visits and counselling sessions, both individual and joint (one for the intending parents and the surrogate couple, the other with the intending parents and the egg donor). The men saw a lawyer and the surrogate couple another lawyer. Oranga Tamariki confirmed they were eligible to adopt, and finally ECART reviewed and approved their case.

The process for Steve and Paul and their surrogate and donor held few surprises. Their initial visit to the clinic and careful noting of the process allowed them all to understand and fulfil the needs for ECART. Currently they have frozen embryos and a pregnant surrogate.

Understanding treatment

Learning about the IVF treatment cycle required for an egg donor means men are able to support their egg donor. The IVF cycle aims to create a number of eggs, which are fertilised and grown into day-five embryos. They will be frozen for later use. Male couples are able to use either a personal donor or a clinic egg donor. When using a clinic donor they may not be involved in her treatment, but can be informed about the results as she goes through IVF. Most clinic donors and recipients wish to meet prior to the treatment.

Once approvals have been received from ECART and the fertility doctor has given the egg donor a cycle plan, she is able to proceed. She will be guided by her nurse through the process of using hormone injections to stimulate her ovaries to make a number of eggs. During this time she will be monitored by blood tests and scans of her ovaries. When the eggs are mature enough she will undergo an egg collection and the eggs will move to the laboratory. Sometime later that day the sperm will be put with the eggs, and the next day fertilisation will be checked. At this point the egg donor's job is done. She will have to wait for a period and then she can use contraception as normal in her life.

The scientists will follow the growth of the fertilised eggs into embryos, and at day five will assess them for freezing. They will only freeze embryos that are likely to have a chance of forming a pregnancy.

In New Zealand there is a three-month quarantine of the embryos before they can be placed into the surrogate; this is to ensure the health of the surrogate is not compromised. The freezing in quarantine will eliminate any infectious issues that may not have been picked up in testing, and so protect the health of the surrogate.

Placement of the embryo into the uterus of the surrogate is a simple procedure and an exciting time, as a pregnancy test nine days later will tell the surrogate and men whether they have been lucky enough to begin a pregnancy.

Pregnancy and birth

The men will be able to tap into one of the many websites that detail how a baby forms to follow the development of the baby in the uterus. These websites are great to follow on a weekly basis, and provide some information about the impact of pregnancy on the mother. The men will need further information on the emotional impact of pregnancy as well as the hormonal and bodily changes that affect her throughout the pregnancy. This information will help the men support her appropriately, especially if they have regular caring communication with their surrogate.

As for all parents, the birth of their child is a wondrous time for these men—one that they had worked hard towards but were often too scared to hope for. As part of the ECART application they will have had a planning discussion about the birth with the surrogate parents. The men will hopefully attend an antenatal course through one of the providers in their area. This will mean they can feel knowledgeable about the process of birth and about ways they can contribute to helping their birth mother. It may also give them support and information about managing a newborn baby.

Post-birth

For the birth mother the three months or so following birth are still connected to the pregnancy. She will likely be feeling a blend of joy at having been able to give these men a child and some grief as her body responds to birth and is prepared for a baby. This does not mean she wants the child, but her body will take time to settle down and her emotions will also settle. The birth mother will have to register the child's birth under her (and, if relevant, her partner's) names.

The men will need to be aware the birth parents will want contact with them and the child. Having lived with the baby for the gestation, the birth parents are unlikely to cope well with an abrupt absence of the child. They will want any existing children to meet the child and to have cuddles and slowly separate. The child will have a special place in their lives. If there is a physical distance between the residences of the two couples, the men would do well to stay a little while in the town of birthing and allow their surrogate to get used to the baby being out of her life.

Part of the IVF Surrogacy Adoption approval allows the men to parent the child from birth. At this point they are not the full guardians, although they can make decisions on medical issues. At 10 working days the men can apply for an interim adoption order and have guardianship of the child. It is not until the final adoption order that they can get a birth certificate with their names as parents and apply for a passport for the child.

Of help to many new parents are 'coffee groups'. These may form through Plunket services or through antenatal groups. In some areas there are special groups for men as full-time parents. Information around this may be found on social media or through local people.

Counselling

Counselling is a required part of using donated sperm or eggs, and it is a good opportunity to explore these issues and the implications of using a donor.

When a person or couple attend counselling they will talk about the HART Act and its implications, and are helped to understand the requirements. While a number of people think perhaps they won't tell their children of the donation or will tell them when they are older, same-gender couples do not have this option, since there are only either eggs or sperm within the couple. They need to be prepared for their child's questions as a preschooler about mothers, fathers and donors.

Clinic donors can choose to donate to several families, although this may vary with different clinics. This means that with the donor's own children, it is likely there will be a number of half-siblings. The implications of this for the future need to be unwrapped, including knowing of the support that can be accessed from the clinic to ensure half-siblings don't become a couple. Ultimately if all the donor-conceived young people know they have a donor and they share this information with their new boyfriend or girlfriend, then they will quickly ascertain this themselves and take steps to see if they share a donor.

Counselling also considers the waiting time for treatment. When using a personal donor there is a quarantine time for the sperm or the embryos to be frozen before they can be used. This quarantine is a safety margin for any infectious issues that may not be identified but can be resolved by freezing. For clinic donors the waiting time is because of the demand for donor sperm, and this will be discussed. When the woman approaches the clinic in her late thirties or early forties, she may not be able to wait long for donor sperm.

Counselling helps people understand more about the people who are happy to donate, and may help the recipients identify what is important to them in selecting a donor. They can talk about the type of information they receive in the profiles they use to choose their donor.

For male couples the need to do surrogacy as well as using a donor means further counselling. As previously discussed, ECART approves surrogacy on case-by-case applications and requires significant counselling. This is to ensure all parties understand the implications of surrogacy (see 'Chapter 15: Surrogacy').

Things to think about

- You may have a wait for the treatment. How can you best use this time to prepare?
- Who will be useful to talk with?
- You may not be entitled to Ministry of Health-funded treatment. Ensure you get a cost estimate from the clinic so you can financially prepare for treatment.
- If you are planning to use a personal donor, consider the role you would like them to play in your lives, keeping the future needs of the child in mind.
- For most same-gender relationships using IVF there are more embryos made than you can use—think this through. While there is no rush to do anything with them, ask the clinic what the options are.

- Not everyone becomes a parent. What resources do you have to deal with this possibility?
- Parental leave is available for parents who adopt a child. Some parental leave is also available to the birth mother.

Things that may be helpful

- Seeking information through sources that are applicable to New Zealand. There are TV documentaries, FertilityNZ as the consumer group has some information, and VARTA (Victorian Assisted Reproductive Treatment Authority) and the UK group The Donor Conception Network have information appropriate to using a donor and helping children understand.
- Finding other people who have undergone this treatment and learning from them.
- Being realistic about the timeframe as there are often delays and unexpected issues within the process. This is often the case when an ethical application is needed and

both an egg donor and a surrogate are to be treated.

- Knowing the treatment process and the cost.

Chapter 12

Using a donor—eggs and sperm

The use of a donor brings fertility treatment to another level—there is another person involved in making the baby. The move to use another person's gametes requires knowledge of the implications and consideration of how these implications will affect all people in the family. Along with understanding the implications, recipients and donors need to know the law, the HART Act 2004, and how it affects donations.

Often called third-party reproduction, the use of donor eggs or donor sperm brings another dimension to family building: the lifetime input from the donor's DNA in the children of the family. Many people are able to accommodate this and raise their children to be confident adults who understand their genetic origins and their family circumstances. There are a few who do not share the information with their young people and then have difficult scenarios when their young adults find out. Young people, with their use of social media and tools such as Ancestry.com, can find out about the donation relatively easily—this has a significant impact on their trust and relationship with their parents.

Amelia

Amelia was aware her parents had used a sperm donor but not of who he was. The donation had taken place before the law requiring donors to be available for contact. While using an ancestry website, she was astonished to find she had a close genetic relative—a man who said he was available to be contacted.

The reality of this took her by surprise, and eventually she told her mother of the development. Her mother was concerned about her father's reaction, but he encouraged her to email this man and ask if he had been a donor.

Things progressed quite quickly from there. Dave (the donor) wanted the meeting to happen at the clinic, and for Amelia to tell him her questions prior to the meeting. He did the same for her.

The meeting was relatively brief, as it transpired Amelia wanted answers to her questions and to meet Dave but no more. She was quite protective of her dad and did not want that relationship challenged. Dave would have been open to future contact but that has not happened.

When considering looking for a donor, the recipients are often clear about what they, as potential parents, need and want. This is their choice and finding an appropriate donor is generally positive for them and their children. Central to deciding the method of finding a donor should be the welfare of the children they hope to parent. Both the recipients' choice of a donor and the way the parents help their children understand the donation are important. Children and young people do best when parents are open and honest with them about their use of donor gametes and answer the young people's questions as they arise.

The decision to use a donor affects relationships differently. Heterosexual couples may find it is the recommended way for them to have children. There is grief as they accept the loss of being the full genetic parents of their child; they need to accept they will be using the gametes of only one potential parent. For same-gender couples and single people there is foreknowledge and acceptance they will need gametes from a donor. This creates a different feeling about the need for a donor.

Grief

For heterosexual people, being told they will need to use donor eggs or donor sperm requires time and consideration so they can accept and welcome this as their means of becoming parents. Their relationship will need reassurance and re-balancing as the couple discuss the loss of one set of their genes in their potential child. It is important to have this discussion prior to beginning treatment with a donor as there is grief for both parties in the loss of the genes. For the person who is able to contribute their genetic material there is the loss of seeing the person they love, and choose to be with, in their children. For the partner who will have no genetic connection to the child the loss of seeing themselves physically in their child, and providing their genetic inheritance to the child, needs to be discussed. Talking about this grief helps with the acceptance of the loss of the genetic input and with success in bonding with the child. Remember that parenting well is an action and not dependent on genetic material.

Same-gender couples bring an awareness they will need someone of the other gender to contribute eggs or sperm. They are most likely to approach treatment with excitement and anticipation rather than grief. The big consideration is how they will find this donor and what they hope to have in a donor in terms of characteristics—physical, personality and abilities.

Similarly, single people may have had to work through the grief at not partnering with someone to help them raise a child. This is balanced by the gratefulness that they can be a parent. The sense of aloneness may arise again as they talk about using a donor, and especially a clinic donor who they will have limited information about.

The law

In New Zealand, donations are regulated by the Human Assisted Reproductive Technology Act 2004 (the HART Act). This Act sets the rules for all reproductive technologies—it advises the clinics about which activities are permitted (such as IVF) and which they must apply to the ethics committee case-by-case to do (such as surrogacy and donor embryos), and also what is forbidden (such as sex-selection in all but a few circumstances). Other countries like Australia and the United Kingdom have similar laws.

Section 3 of the HART Act covers donations. Donations of eggs and sperm where one party is still the genetic parent are established procedures and permitted, but the use of donor embryos or using both donated eggs and donated sperm require case-by-case applications to the ethics committee for approval.

In New Zealand, as in Australia and the United Kingdom, there is no anonymous donation—the laws state that young people have a right to their genetic information. Donors and prospective parents are told of this and the reasons why it is in the child's best interests to know of their genetic origins. To this end certain information is collected from the donor, and this is available for the young person or their guardian as non-identifying information prior to age 18. At 18 years, or in some situations earlier, the young person can seek the identity of their donor and will be given it. Identifying information is available on request to a parent or guardian before the child turns 18.

When the donor child is born their birth is recorded on the Donor Register held by Births, Deaths and Marriages. The information held is the name, date of birth, place of birth and current address of the donor-conceived child, the parent(s) and the donor. This is a closed register available to the young person, or their guardians in some circumstances, at 18.

Donors are not paid—all donations are altruistic, although clinics have an arrangement covering a small level of expenses related to the donation, such as mileage, GP appointments and other expenses directly related to the donation. Each organisation deals with this in their own way. All parties need to be aware of the expenses so they can plan in advance, particularly when it is a personal donation from a family member or friend.

There are other considerations before using a donor.

Personal donor or clinic donor?

The decision whether to use a personally recruited donor or a clinic-recruited donor needs to be carefully thought through. Both have advantages and disadvantages, and where people have the choice they need to choose based on the future wellbeing of the child. It is the child who will live with this decision, so carefully weighing up how this is best for a child in a family is important.

Often the need to use a donor follows other unsuccessful treatment, and this requires time to firstly grieve and then to talk about issues such as how important a genetic connection to the child is for them. This may vary—some women feel carrying the pregnancy is enough of a connection to the child for them; others would prefer to use a sister or cousin they are close to. For men the genetic connection may be very important—this can be to do with their faith or keeping the family name and inheritance of the genetic line alive. For many of the people needing a donation, finding a personal donor they feel confident to use is close to impossible. The relief at finding a clinic donor who they feel is appropriate to them outweighs the need for a genetic connection.

At the beginning of this decision the recipients need to gather information.

They need to understand the implications of using a personal donor or a clinic-recruited donor, and also the availability of donors. Counselling is required before being able to use a donor, and this is a great opportunity to gather information to help make the decision.

A donor brings different DNA into a family, and it is important that the couple recognise the implications of having third-party genes within the family. The considerations include the relationship the recipients wish to have with their donor; the relationship of the donor with the donor children; who they may tell about the donation; and the impact this telling may have on those people's relationship with the child. It is also important to think about the wellbeing of the child within that family unit. Will the child have a sense of belonging and acceptance if physically and emotionally they are very different from the family in which they live? There are no rights or wrongs in answering these questions, as families and people vary and can accommodate different things.

The decision whether to look for a personal donor and known genes or wait on the clinic list for a non-identified donor is clear for some people but less clear for others. Some people are easily able to think of a family member or friend who may be willing to donate. These people may need some ideas about how to ask that person to consider donation and what they are asking them to go through. The recipients and their potential donor will discuss their plans for talking and telling the donor's children as well as the potential donor child. There will be some need to manage the sharing of the donor information given they may have friends or family in common.

Albert and Lily

Albert and Lily (their English names) were told they needed an egg donor and that the clinic did not have any Chinese egg donors available, nor did Chinese women offer to donate eggs to strangers very often. Fortunately Lily's sister had had successful IVF and offered to donate.

Albert and Lily had decided they would not tell anyone about the donation as they were fearful about how their family and friends would react to the information. They expected criticism and feared rejection of the child.

A robust discussion took place in counselling where their fears were gently unwrapped. They were very concerned about both sets of parents accepting the child. When asked about their parents as people they assured the counsellor they were very accepting people who had adapted well to the culture of this country. They talked about the parents' grief that they did not have children. Lily's parents had her sister's child, but Albert's parents had no grandchildren to carry the family into the future. Lily and Albert were able to recognise that Lily's parents might feel reassured since her sister was the donor. They decided that since Albert's sperm was being used to create the child his parents would see the child as from their family.

The couple decided to begin by telling Lily's parents, who it turned out were quite able to support the use of the sister as donor. The parents asked they tell no one and especially not the child about the donation, but the sisters were clear the children needed to know and they wanted to be truthful. They agreed this would be 'in-family information'.

Albert's parents struggled a bit more with the information, as they had struggled with IVF when told of that. Their desire to have a grandchild eventually won them over, although when they saw Lily pregnant they disregarded the donor information and decided the miracle they had prayed for had happened. The child is a much-adored family member.

This example highlights the capacity of families to come to terms with donations and also how, for some families, the use of a personal donor is preferable. Families will sometimes ask for the donation to be kept secret, but most couples can see the rationale around being honest and respectful to their child. They recognise that children learn about DNA at school, so the child may find out about the donor if they discover their blood group is different from their parents'. This is one example of young people learning of their genetic origins—when they learn from sources other than their parents they generally feel disappointed at the lack of honesty, and trust may be very hard to re-establish.

Puberty is the time when young people are developing their identity and answering questions such as 'Who am I?' At that stage the young person may ask a parent about the donor, and if they are able to say 'It was our friend Shannon', the child who knows the donor is able to incorporate that into their identity development. The young person will at some stage need to explore the social and genetic relationships with the donor and that person's children. As long as parents have an open relationship with their young person and answer their questions, this will managed.

For some people finding a personal donor is not a possibility; when they explore the people in their lives they cannot find a suitable person to ask. These people will seek a clinic-recruited donor. There is likely to be a wait, often long, before a donor is available and there may be only a small choice of donors. Donors are able to give directions about who can use their donation and clinics follow these directions.

Many clinic egg donors and some sperm donors are willing and sometimes keen to meet their recipients before the donation. Egg donors are often geographically close to the recipients, but sperm donations are kept in a central pool, meaning that they may come from across the country and be harder to have contact with prior to the treatment.

The meetings between clinic egg donors and their recipients are an opportunity to get a sense of each other and to plan their contact and information-sharing in the future.

Mia and Tane

Mia and Tane both come from large extended whānau with many cousins around their age. They talked at length about what made a person a good potential donor—healthy, nonsmoker, no recreational drugs, moderate alcohol intake and preferably finished creating their own family. For an egg donor, which is what they needed, the donor must have a normal BMI. Mia stated categorically that her cousins were all out as no one fitted these criteria; Tane had a couple of names of cousins, who Mia ruled out.

They felt they would like to explore a clinic donor, and talked about how for them having contact with the donor in the future was a must. They did not want to be best friends, but did want to be able to call and have a coffee occasionally.

Mia and Tane were lucky: after a wait, a donor was found who also wanted to know the family receiving the donation. This donor directed the clinic as to the sort of people her donation was to go to, and Mia and

Tane fitted well. At the joint meeting the donor and her partner expressed their delight in helping this young couple. They all agreed the children from both families should know of the donation at a young age; no secrets. The donating couple thought this was very important, both because they wanted to be honest and also because they feared the children could meet and develop a romantic attachment in adolescence if they didn't know they were related.

Mia and Tane have two children now, and are bringing them up with full knowledge of the donors and their children, but also with their Māori whakapapa and te reo (Māori language) so they will be confident about their origins in all ways. The two families meet at least once a year to keep contact.

Talking and telling the children

Children and young people deserve respect and honesty from their parents. Children can cope with information about their origins when it is given positively and with love. Ideally they should be brought up with the knowledge that their parent(s) needed a hand to have a child and that the donor provided this help. The first question may be 'What is a donor?' and the answer is simple and honest: 'It is the person who gave us the eggs or sperm to make a baby because we needed help.' Children can cope with this at preschool level, and are likely to ask questions as they grow. Answering them honestly but with simple answers is best. This means that there is not a big confession where the parents are nervous about being rejected or fear adolescent behaviours.

Parents who do not tell children or other significant people in their lives of the donation are generally either ashamed they need a donor or fearful of the reaction. They may worry their children will not see them as proper parents. Research is clear that children who are well parented and loved see those who parent them as their parents regardless of the genetic connection.

It does take extra effort to use a donor and courage to bring children up knowing their genetic origins. It helps if the parents of donor children are able to use positive and supportive language when talking about the donor. This gives the young person a sense of having a likeable donor and having good genes, so if they decide to meet the donor they approach this meeting feeling good about themselves and the donor's role in their lives.

When a child is treated with respect and honesty their identity development is enhanced and they have resilience to cope with life and the variations it brings.

Things to think about

- How important is the genetic connection to you?

- Who would be able to provide the DNA? Do you and your partner agree about this person as a donor?
- How would the child feel about meeting this person (the personal donor)?
- You will need to discuss the telling and talking with your children and consider the donor's children as well.
- Who will you tell, what will you say, and when will you say it? Remember if you tell people before treatment, you cannot 'untell'.
- How will your child feel when you tell them you used a clinic donor?
- How will you explain each of these issues to your child?

Things that may be helpful

- Talking with online support groups—in New Zealand there are 'parents of egg-donor children' and 'single parents by choice' groups online. Also search Facebook for groups.
- Seeking out books to read—your clinic may have some you can

borrow. *Inheritance* by Dani Shapiro is a good start. There are also books to help you talk to your children.

- Being aware that online information may be written by people who have had treatment under very different circumstances—overseas clinics that only do anonymous donation, clinics that pay their donors significant money.
- Finding someone who has had a child by donation and talking with them.
- Sharing with someone you trust so you can process this information as you go along.
- Looking at the UK Donor Conception Network's resources, or those of VARTA, the Victoria Assisted Reproductive Authority.
- Watching the webinars FertilityNZ has on their donor and surrogacy network.

Chapter 13

Donor sperm

Donations of sperm were one of the earliest fertility interventions. The inseminations were offered in a range of medical practices before fertility clinics existed, such as some GP practices and urology clinics—places where a lack of sperm might be noted. The recommendation to couples was to have intercourse that evening and not to tell the child about the donation, as they could not be sure about paternity.

The sperm came from a variety of places—students were often offered the opportunity to donate, particularly medical students, and understood that no records were kept so they would be anonymous. There was little thought to the implications for the young people born as a result of the donation. By the 1980s there was more awareness about the needs of children, and donors in the clinics were encouraged to be available in the future. Many of them were able to appreciate that the young people born as a result of donor sperm might have health or identity issues that compromised their wellbeing. These donors were open to being approached by the clinic for information and sometimes contact.

When men provide sperm for the creation of families by donation it is a generous gift of potential life. Donors nowadays often know someone who has needed a donation to become a parent, and many of them know the joy of parenting. They are asked to consider carefully the implications of this gift for all parties, including their own children. The people who choose or need to use donor sperm for family creation also have to weigh up the implications. This chapter is an opportunity to consider situations where donor sperm is an appropriate treatment, and the impact of using donor sperm, and to provide an opportunity to begin the thinking about the choices that need to be made.

There are a number of situations where donated sperm is needed for heterosexual couples. Same-gender female couples and single women also require donor sperm to parent. The process of getting a donor is similar for all parties; the emotional issues around using donor sperm vary considerably.

Heterosexual couples

When a couple discover the man has no sperm, or the sperm cannot be used perhaps because of a genetic condition, they first have to deal with the grief and loss of his lack of sperm and sometimes his change in perception of himself. The couple will also have to come to terms with the fact they will not see his attributes portrayed directly in their child. Sometimes a man may know or suspect something is awry, but for many the news from the doctor is shattering and challenges the man's whole view of himself as a man. This may cause a variety of feelings—anger, deep sadness, insecurity, questioning of his manliness, and the fear of telling others or them finding out about his lack of sperm.

The initial shock creates a very hard time. At the beginning the man may not be able to believe this is correct information or accept reassurance from his partner that she is there for him and they will get through this together. Accepting his partner's reassurance that she loves him for him is important. She may need to repeat this and show love, caring and intimacy while he learns to accept his lack of sperm. He may feel guilt that he cannot give his partner a child, and some men feel their worth as a man is compromised. Shock and denial have a purpose in ensuring the man is not overwhelmed by the information. These emotions are mostly short-lived and gradual acceptance of this truth will happen. During this time the man may not wish to be around others, and particularly not friends with children.

While this is happening the woman will also feel distress and disbelief, and will be disappointed to know she will not have a child with the DNA of the man she loves. These strong feelings are often stored or dealt with away from her partner so she can stand firm to support him.

While the shock of learning about the lack of sperm will take a while to accept, there are some things that help us stay grounded and able to function. These will be different for everybody, but may include exercising or going for a walk together. Physical movement helps emotions move forward. Seeking places that provide comfort, like the beach, the bush, a high point with a lovely view or a walk that is very familiar, is reassuring that other things have not changed. If you like swimming, being in the water and being buoyed up by it may provide relief. Some people like to listen to music, others find solace in preparing and eating favourite foods. These activities are all sensory and allow us to focus on caring for ourselves. Going back to normal work routines and feeling competent at work will generally help regain the balance of yourself as a person.

Josie and Glen

Glen had withdrawn from Josie after the specialist told him of his lack of sperm. He seemed to be doing his usual routine of work and activities, but when Josie talked with him he often did not respond and she felt he had not heard her. She was concerned she was losing the desire to keep trying to talk and sort this out. Then his work rang her and expressed concern about him, and she decided to try again.

That evening she asked him to come for a walk along the waterfront. This was an activity they enjoyed a couple of times a week. Glen tried to call off, but she told him clearly she needed him to do this for her.

He was definitely a reluctant starter so she waited until they were quite a way from the car before she talked. She told him how she felt when she was not allowed to help him—she loved him dearly and he was the most important person in her life. She told him she could live without kids but did not want to live without him. With tears streaming down her face, she asked him to talk about what was in his head.

As she realised he, too, was crying, she suggested they go into the sand dunes for some privacy and they sat and cried together. The words slowly came out about his sense he should let her go so she could partner with someone else, and his despair at that thought.

Josie realised how damaged he felt, but at least now he was talking to her so they had a chance to sort it out. She made sure they did comforting things together over the next few days and weeks, and she reassured him of her love through caring actions and a few comments. When they got back to talking about the lack of sperm, Glen was able to talk about it as part of him and not the whole of him. He was beginning to accept that she saw it as their problem, rather than his problem.

This is often quite a short stage and the couple regains functioning and getting through daily life. When they are ready they are likely to begin talking about what next and exploring how far they are prepared to go to be parents. The couple are likely to touch on donor sperm, adoption, 'home for life' (where the child has been removed from his or her parents and the couple have guardianship in conjunction with Oranga Tamariki until the child is 18 years old) and being child-free. These are appropriate issues to consider before making a decision. Seeking more information about some of these is important so the discussions can be informed.

When the man cannot use his sperm, the specialist at the clinic will score the couple for public funding, and a good many couples will be eligible to have their treatment paid for by the government. Counselling is a requirement for accessing donor sperm in both funded and private cycles. The clinic counsellor holds a lot of information about donor sperm, and is able to help the couple become informed for effective decision-making. The counsellor will also be able to tell them where to seek information about other ways of parenting if they wish to research these as well.

Accessing donor sperm can happen through the clinic donor lists or by finding a personal donor. As will become apparent at the clinic, there are long waiting lists for clinic donors whereas a personally recruited donor can be ready in about six months.

Personally recruited donors

Finding a personally recruited donor requires some consideration of the people in your world. Sometimes the man would like some of his genetic material in the child and is lucky enough to have a brother who they like and feel able to ask. Other times it's a cousin, or some men have a friend with whom they have a close friendship with to allow this request. Taking time to think about how being a donor and recipient may change your relationship with this man and his partner and children is important. The donating man will have a genetic connection to your children and any existing or future children will be half-siblings to your children. Often the two couples can move to a heightened level of friendship, caring and support.

After deciding to use a personal donor and deciding who to approach, perhaps the hardest task is how to ask the friend/brother/cousin to consider donating. It takes a lot of courage to ask if someone would consider sharing their sperm. In fact you are paying them a significant compliment, as you are essentially saying that he has the sort of genes you would like to see in your child. Deciding what to say and trusting that the man will be respectful with the information of your infertility shows a confidence and belief in him and his partner.

Josie and Glen (continued)

While Glen talked about his infertility it was quite a long time before he was ready to talk about donor sperm. One day he abruptly said he did not want to be a dad unless he knew the genes of the child. Josie knew he must have been thinking about a donor and just now had found a way to talk with her. She asked him to tell her what he was thinking. He said he felt his cousin

Billy was the person he trusted most and he wondered if he might donate. He thought Billy's partner, Rochelle, would agree, but he wanted to know how Josie felt about it.

It took Josie quite by surprise as she had thought he might not get to the point of considering a donor. She asked him to talk more about how this happened, and wondered if he would take the lead in talking to Billy.

Glen took Billy fishing and in the course of the day asked him to consider donation. Billy talked with Rochelle and then called to say they wanted to help. The four of them then had a talk about how they would manage this now and in the future. They talked with their fertility clinic and stepped into the process.

At the time Josie told her story, they were just about to begin inseminations with the donor sperm. She shared her story to help other women support their partner at this difficult time.

PS: It took three inseminations before Josie and Glen became pregnant, and they are now parents to a son and hope in time to have another child. Josie and Glen and Billy and Rochelle talk with a shared pride of their achievement. They have chosen not to share this with their families at this point.

As part of the preparation for using donor sperm, each couple needs to consider the implications of the donation for them and their children. Together the two couples will discuss and reach mutual decisions about many things. These include who they are going to tell about the donation, at what ages they will help the children understand, and the relationships they are creating and how they will manage them over time.

Children born as a result of a personally recruited donor are generally advantaged as they will have access to the donor as they grow up and become curious about their genetic information. While clinic donors may feel like the easier, or perhaps only, option for some couples, their children may only have non-identifying information until they are 18 years.

Clinic-recruited donors

Couples are likely to choose to use a clinic-recruited donor if they do not know anyone they feel is suitable to be a personally recruited donor. Clinic-recruited donors share extensive personal and family medical information with the specialist, and undergo counselling prior to their sperm being accepted onto the programme. This provides some safeguards for recipients.

There are factors to understand and think about when using a clinic donor. Firstly, the length of the waiting list is generally a disappointment as people often feel ready to have treatment quite quickly. When your turn comes to choose a donor, you will have access to a limited number of profiles of non-identifying information about the donors and only sometimes will there be a baby photograph. Your donor is likely to have donated to create a number of families (check with your clinic about their rules on this), so your children are likely to have a number of half-siblings in other families as well as the donor's children. The donor will have given family and personal medical health information as well as mental health information to the specialist, and some genetic testing is done.

Having considered and decided these aspects are acceptable to you, you can be reassured that the men who wish to donate are generally generous and have a genuine wish to help families have a child or children.

It is important to understand the HART Act in relation to using a donor, as it states that children have a right to their genetic information. This information is kept within a Donor Register held by Births, Deaths and Marriages. It is filled out when the child is born and held in a closed register for the child to access at 18 years, or under some circumstances earlier. Parents can access it from the child's birth.

Same-gender female couples and single women

Single women and same-gender female couples have many similarities with heterosexual couples. They have the same considerations about the choice of a clinic-recruited donor or a personally recruited donor. A big difference is they arrive at the clinic knowing they need donor sperm to have a child, so they have a different emotional position.

For single women there may be grief and loss at not having found the right person to form a long-term relationship and have children with, combined with the sadness caused by needing to involve another person, who they may not know, in the creation of their child. These emotions may be felt alongside the gratefulness they feel to have donor sperm available to them.

Kylie

Kylie had come out of a long-term relationship with Wiremu about 18 months before coming to the clinic.

The relationship ended because she wanted a child and he had previous children and thought that was enough.

Kylie's sadness about the relationship and not having a father for her child dominated the first counselling session. She came back to counselling as she wanted to work on using a donor—she thought working through this would give her a sense of having a future with a child.

Kylie was 38 and understood the impact of age and the length of the clinic donor waiting list, so she decided to consider a personal donor. Having collected a lot of information about treatments and personal donors, Kylie felt she had enough information to sort out her options.

Three months later Wiremu appeared at counselling. He explained that they had decided that if she was to have a donor he would be happy to do this. The child would know he was the donor and who its half-siblings were, but he would not be the father. Hence doing the donation through the clinic.

Both Kylie and Wiremu wanted the child to know its whakapapa. They hoped it would be nestled in the two families and whānau, with Kylie as the child's parent.

Same-gender female couples have the person they love alongside of them, and they too feel glad they can use donor sperm. These couples look forward to being parents and often feel ready in their lives and relationship to be parents. Some may be frustrated by the long waiting list for a clinic donor. Others come to the clinic aware of the wait and use the time to prepare for the parenthood they hope to achieve when the sperm is available.

The choice of a personally recruited donor or a clinic-recruited donor is a big decision. When thinking about a personally recruited donor the women need to think about the ongoing relationship they will have with the man in the future and his relationship with the child. By having agreement on how all people see these relationships evolving, they have made a good start. It is an advantage to be able to communicate easily and discuss the needs of the child. These change as the child ages, and will continue to need to be met.

Women are aware of the importance of feeling confident they have a chosen a donor who their child will like if they meet him in the future. When using a donor who has been through the clinic process they can also feel safe that their donor has been assessed as being appropriate to donate sperm and understands the implications of the donation, including his lack of responsibilities and rights towards the child.

Some single women and same-gender female couples have sought male donors on donor websites. Sometimes this works well. In New Zealand there have been, and possibly still are, men who do not respect the agreements they and the women create prior to creating a child. These men cause a lot of concern for the women who used their sperm. The parents worry their child has the genes of this man who they no longer like or trust. Some of these cases have ended in court battles causing anger, anxiety and high economic costs for the recipient family as they seek trespass and non-contact prohibitions.

Clinic-recruited donors

Making a choice about using a clinic-recruited donor ensures the donor will have been through a series of checks to ensure he should be a good donor. He will have been checked for infectious diseases and have had some genetic testing included. His sperm will have been assessed. The specialist will have done a personal and family physical and mental health history, and the donor will have had counselling with his partner to ensure they understand the legal, social and genetic implications of donating sperm. When choosing to use a clinic donor it is reassuring to know the donor has been through a relatively comprehensive process.

Much of the counselling before using a donor is information-giving, then discussing how this information will impact on you and your life. Deciding who to share the donor information with as early as possible will be an advantage down the line when the child begins to ask questions.

Prior to choosing a donor, you need to think about some of the characteristics you hope to find. When the profiles are in front of you, you may need to choose which attributes are a priority. Always remember that half of your child's DNA will come from you.

Managing who to tell what about the donor is important. New Zealand is a series of relatively interconnected communities, and people may be able, or think they are able, to identify your donor from his profile. Being discreet with this information will ensure that when your child needs it you are the person who shares it.

When the children of female couples and single women reach about three years old, they notice other children have a father. They are likely to ask you about their lack of a father. You can help them understand they do not have a father but they do have a donor instead—the man who helped you have a child. Using the correct language is important, as children observe and develop concepts of what roles, both emotional and activity-based, a father has in children's lives. Donors seldom want to be involved with the child. They have their own families in which they are parents.

As they mature, the young people may need more information about their donor than the non-identifying profiles provide. They may feel different from you, their parent(s), or very curious about the person who provided half of their DNA. Donors take the wellbeing of the young people they have helped create seriously, and are generally approachable about finding a way to help. It is nevertheless important to realise that donors' lives move forward over the years and their circumstances may change.

A useful tool is to help the young person identify what it is they would like to know, and to check in with the counsellor about the ways in which this information can be accessed. Sometimes an email can be sent via the counsellor for the donor to respond to. The donor may even be willing to send a photo of himself at the young person's age. Other times the counsellor can ask the donor the questions and transmit the answers. Certainly if the young person wishes to meet the donor, then the counsellor will need to make contact with the donor to see about his availability. While a portion of donors are happy to meet, others might have had a change in life circumstances since they donated—a new partner who is not supportive, or a change of residence within New Zealand or overseas—and may not be available to meet. Some wish to wait until the child is close to adulthood at 18 to meet.

There are seldom situations where the young person cannot get the information needed in some shape or form, but parents need to be wary of raising the donor child's hopes before they know of the possibilities available.

Things to think about

For heterosexual couples

- What is manliness? Is it about fathering a child or being a good person?
- What makes a man a good father?
- How can you deal with any anger that presents itself?
- How important is it to you to have a genetic connection to your children?
- Is the ability to love dictated by genes? (Do you love your pets?) Do you think you can love a child who is dependent on you but not linked to you genetically?
- If you are the woman in a heterosexual couple, you may need someone safe to help you with your own feelings while you support the man you love.
- If you are a man in need of donor sperm, you may feel guilty if your partner has to undergo treatment because of you. How does she feel about this?

For all using donor sperm

- What are some things you might like in your donor?
- Who can you trust to tell who will respect this information and not share it with others?
- How can you manage the wait and prepare for treatment?
- What donor terminology would be most helpful to the child as it grows up?
- Children do not really understand eggs and sperm until they get towards puberty—consider what simple explanations you can provide for them.
- Daughters often want more information than sons. How do you manage this difference?
- Donors have no rights or responsibilities for the children, but they do have to be identifiable when the young person is 18 or if the Family Court is involved at 16 or 17. Many donors are happy to answer questions and maybe meet before that.

Things that might be helpful

- Reading carefully about others' experiences—New Zealand, Australia and the United Kingdom have many similarities in donors' stories. The Victoria Assisted Reproductive Treatment Authority (VARTA) in Australia and the Donor Conception Network in the United Kingdom are among other groups that produce useful reading.
- Joining a New Zealand support group on Facebook.
- Talking with your support network if appropriate.
- Making contact with the FertilityNZ Donor Conception and Surrogacy network.
- Practising self-care (see section entitled "Maintaining wellbeing – Resilience in times of waiting").

Chapter 14

Donor eggs

Being told by the specialist that using donor eggs is your only way to become a parent takes time for any woman or couple to accept. As with donor sperm, the knowledge that another person will bring DNA to the child you are parenting requires a move from wishing to have a child who reflects both of you, to accepting that parenting is the goal you want to achieve. For many couples this transition takes a while; for others having a solution is a relief, and they welcome the treatment and work to understand the implications.

Donation of eggs occurs when a fertile woman undergoes an IVF cycle to gift her eggs to another woman to create a family. It is an act of generosity that some women are able to manage.

For donors

Undergoing IVF is a big step to undertake to help others have a family. IVF is a significant event, and the donor will be encouraged to think about and understand the process of IVF before she makes the decision to donate. Donors need to consider the implications of sharing their genes and the connection this will create for them and their children.

Among the implications a donor is asked to consider is her relationship with the recipients. A donation changes a relationship by creating a genetic connection within it, and this will require discussion and management. Personal donors are required to have a joint meeting with the recipients to ensure they discuss the management of the donation both for now and for the future of these two families.

A clinic donor is able to direct the clinic with some wishes about who she donates to. Commonly donors give the clinic directions on some of the following—meeting and having some contact, ethnicity, beliefs, mental health, previous children and sometimes the age of the recipient. Clinic donors frequently wish to meet their recipients, and having done this the donor may wish to have some contact with them to hear about the birth of the child.

Stacey

Stacey had thought about being an egg donor since she read an article in a women's magazine. When she had had her own children, she decided to follow through with this desire. She came to the clinic and fulfilled all the requirements of egg donation, then was linked with a recipient couple. She asked to meet them, and when they walked in it was a woman she had briefly met at a party. Stacey was not comfortable as this felt too close, so decided not to proceed.

Another link was made with new recipients, and this time they were, as Stacey wished, unknown to her at the meeting. She liked these people and was pleased when they told her they wanted their children to grow up knowing about the donation and if possible to know her. She asked them if she could contact them directly to share results throughout the IVF. The couple agreed and proceeded to offer her support during treatment.

They have regular contact and, although they do not mix socially, celebrate the milestones of the donor-created children together.

Personal donors also need to consider IVF and the implications for themselves, their partner and their children of sharing their genes. They need to consider the relationship between them and their recipients as it is now, and how they perceive it may be in the future as the children want information. This will be talked through firstly in their individual counselling session. A joint counselling session is required before treatment, to enable the parties to discuss the management of this donation together and look towards the wellbeing of the children—both the donor's children and the hoped-for recipients' children. Discussion will include the timing of talking and telling the donor's children of the donation. The language each person uses will help the children define the relationship. For example, using 'donor' rather than 'donor mother' helps both the donor's children and the new child be clear about where they fit in both families. Generally the donor's children will be older and may know before the recipient's children are ready for the information. The donor often tells her existing children she is donating her eggs, but not always who she is donating to.

Agreement about managing this is important as the recipient child needs to be told by its parents rather than getting a story from the donor's children or another person.

For recipients

People who need donor eggs have much to consider prior to launching themselves into this treatment. Initially there may be a wave of grief that a woman will need another fertile woman to help them have a child. The woman may have a sense of failure that her body cannot provide the eggs for her child. Sadness about not seeing the physical characteristics she likes about herself in her children should be discussed.

Her partner, while supporting her to work through this, has his own grief at not seeing the woman he loves in their children. The physical characteristics will not be present, but as children grow they take on the attitudes, values and mannerisms of their parents.

One of the ways people move to acceptance of using a donor is to evaluate how much they want to be parents. If the desire to parent is greater than the need to use the woman's gametes then it is easier to accept the donation and the children that result.

Most people know of someone who has a step-parent or has been adopted—some type of parenting where there are different genes. These are often successful relationships. They are successful because the parents manage the environment in which the child grows. The child feels loved and learns about their family's relationships and values. Genes are important and need to be considered. A couple raising a donor child will provide one set of genes and all of the environment, and so be the majority influences in the young person's life.

Being pregnant with a child created by donation can be challenging for some people. The delight in finally knowing they will be parents may have the shadow of the donation behind it.

Shannon and Ryan

Shannon and Ryan were finally pregnant after using eggs donated by Shannon's cousin. They had discussed this donation within their whānau and it was supported by both families. Shannon however had another wave of loss and grief as she thought about the pregnancy, and Ryan seemed unable to help her through this.

In counselling we acknowledged the loss of her genetic material and the impact this had on her. We talked about the genes she was getting from her cousin and recognised they were family genes. We considered uterine impact on the child and how the hormones of her body were influencing the development of the baby inside her.

Her whānau had accepted the donation by likening it to a whāngai relationship. This had made Shannon anxious as she knew of a whāngai child whose genetic and legal parents took him back. In counselling we discussed the registration and birth certificate, reassuring Shannon that she and Ryan would be the legal parents to their baby.

While this was very reassuring and gave her answers that she shared with her whānau, the biggest comfort occurred after the birth of her baby when her cousin came to see her and talked about Shannon's child and how she did not feel at all maternal towards the child. Shannon was excited to share this with the counsellor.

Sharing information about the donation

There are a number of ways a couple may share information about the donation. The biggest consideration in this is the children created by the donation. Their sense of themselves will depend on the honesty of their parents and the care they take to help the child feel good about their genetic background.

For some couples the news they have a donor is so exciting they tell all their family and friends about it. These couples will need to be open and honest with their children from the beginning. It is important children understand the donation from their parents' point of view rather than hearing from another person. Children are often reluctant to talk with their parents if they feel the conversation will be painful to the parents. This opens up room for misunderstandings.

Carly and Harry

We had told everyone about the donation (but not who the donor was) as soon as we were pregnant. We were so excited. We realised that our family considered this open knowledge to be talked about anytime. So we wrote to our clinic donor and began to get to know her a bit more. When our son was born we asked her if she would consider coming to our celebration and us introducing her as the donor. She was so brave to allow us to do this and our family showed great aroha to her. She and her son have become part of our family now. The boys know they are brothers.

Research literature on adoption and donor sperm, and emerging studies of egg donations, are very clear that children can cope with this knowledge. Children do best when it is knowledge they have always had, rather than acquired from a 'telling' by parents. This means they grow up with a single, stable version of reality and develop an identity that includes this information. As they grow up through puberty and adolescence they may explore this information and include it when they consider the important questions: 'Who am I?', 'What sort of person do I want to be?', 'What made me like I am?'

The fear of telling belongs to the parents. Sometimes the woman is scared she will be seen as inadequate, other times the parents fear the young adolescent will throw the donation back in their face—'You are not my real parent.' Before using a donation you need to make a commitment to respecting your children and helping them understand why you used a donor and how important being parents is to you. Deciding what makes a good parent means determining whether it is the genes or the actions of parenting that create the love, trust and respect between parents and children. One way of doing this is to think about our own lives and remember what was important to us about our parents.

A number of parents decide to tell the child as questions about life are asked, and just build the information into their lives. A general belief for parents who decide to do this is always to answer the questions honestly and to ensure the young person feels free to ask questions. By puberty when they are beginning to answer the question 'Who am I?', young people need to understand their genetic origins.

A few couples, sometimes due to cultural considerations, decide not to tell the child of the donation. Both our law, the HART Act, and the clinics are clear that young people have a right to their genetic information. There are many stories about young people finding out they are donor-created.

Jordan

One morning as I arrived at the clinic to begin the day, I found in the waiting room a couple whose faces were familiar, although I could not name them. They had with them a young man. All were visibly upset.

I invited them into my office and asked them to tell me what was happening for them. It transpired that their son, Jordan, was 16 and had donated blood at school. When he received the letter giving his blood type he knew one of his parents was not his genetic parent (blood types are studied at school). He had confronted his parents that evening and they were all needing help.

The parents went off for a coffee while I talked with Jordan. He told me he was in no doubt about who his mother was; she had been a great mum. He was upset and angry that his parents had not trusted him enough to tell him of the donation.

We talked at length about the fear his parents had about rejection, and how the longer they left it the harder it became to raise the subject. He accepted that, although he felt they now needed to have a good talk.

He invited them back into the room and put his arms around them and told them never to doubt his love, but that they all would now have to work on the trust. They decided they could manage the talk they needed without my help.

Finding an egg donor

As with sperm donation there can be a significant wait for a clinic-recruited egg donor. This causes a good number of women to look into their family and friendship groups to find a personally recruited donor. Sometimes people are lucky enough to have someone close to them offer.

Other women and couples go onto websites that facilitate opportunities for donors and recipients to connect. These connections are still regarded by the clinics as personally recruited, so it is important for both parties to invest some energy into getting to know each other prior to their having the required joint meeting at a clinic.

Another means of finding a donor occurs when the woman or couple create a private section on their Facebook account and ask their family and close friends if they know anyone who might consider being a donor. A number of people have found success this way.

When people have no one suitable to ask to donate, the clinic lists are the next option. When sperm-donation recipient couples who fit the donor's directions come to the top of the waiting list they are able to choose from a number of male donor profiles. In egg donation, the donor selects the recipient couple from their profile, and then they are offered the donor's profile. This occurs because IVF for the donor takes place after the couple is chosen. Most donors are relatively flexible, but they may also have some criteria they want in recipients. Clinics will seek the most appropriate recipients. Following the linking of recipients and donors, the clinic will facilitate the next stages.

A frozen egg bank is in development at one clinic, and this will potentially make eggs more available to recipients. An example of this happens when a donor is likely to produce a large number of eggs—enough for two or more recipients. The coordinators of the egg bank will talk the donors and recipients through the process to see if it matches their needs. Donors will still be able to provide some direction about their recipients.

Some recipients wish to go overseas for egg donation. This is possible at a number of overseas clinics; however, there are few who provide known donors—most are able to give a profile but the donors remain anonymous. The New Zealand law (and also Australian and United Kingdom laws) and the clinics recognise that young people are able to develop best when they have access to their genetic information and the background information about their donor. In the best interests of the child the option of an anonymous donor needs to be chosen warily.

Using an egg donor

When considering egg donation as an option, couples need to think about and discuss how the woman will feel carrying a child who is made from another woman's eggs. For most women, meeting the donor and talking about the donation provides comfort in the feeling they have received eggs from a person they like. Many women recognise they contribute biologically by providing the uterus and environment for the pregnancy. This allows them to feel close to the baby.

The donor provides half of the DNA for the child, and for most people having a donor who is a relatively good 'fit' with them looks-wise is best. It makes life with the child easier as they are not constantly having to explain to other people how they have become the parents to the child. It is in the child's best interests to feel as if they belong within this family and do not need to explain the family to curious outsiders.

Men will sometimes feel a bit uncomfortable with their sperm being used to fertilise an egg from the donor. When using IVF this takes place within the laboratory and it is not until an embryo is formed that it is placed into the recipient woman's uterus. This distance is useful in helping deal with the strangeness of fertilising another woman's eggs.

Meeting a clinic-recruited donor is possible, and many of the donors wish to meet. If the donor wishes to meet, then only recipients who are happy to do so will be considered. These meetings are challenging for both parties, as they want to present well and be liked. Many donors will ask for a small amount of information after the birth of children so they can tell their children about half-siblings.

Sometimes donors will produce a lot of eggs. This may be predicted by their AMH and other tests, or it may be unexpected. Once a donor and recipient are linked and these eggs have sperm put with them, the decisions about them belong to the recipients. Having too many embryos may mean that after finishing their family they have to make the decision to dispose of or (if the donor is willing and consents) donate the embryos. There is a maximum of two families with full genetic siblings in New Zealand, which means children with the same eggs and sperm can only exist in the recipient couple's family and one embryo-donation-created family. Disposal of embryos can be challenging, as they have taken so much effort to achieve. Clinics are happy to dispose of embryos for people; equally, if the couple wish to take them home to have a ceremony and dispose of them themselves this can be facilitated.

Egg donors can provide a solution to childlessness. Approaching the use of a donor needs thought and discussion—with the best interests of any resulting child at the forefront.

Things to think about

- There is grief in hearing that your own eggs will not form a child; feeling sad and resentful is normal.
- Failure is a common feeling when a woman is not able to use her own eggs, so you need to be compassionate with yourself. Recognise that while not having successful eggs is huge, your body does look after you in so many other ways.
- Most women who need donor eggs are able to carry the child through a pregnancy.
- Which is more important if you have to choose—being a parent or only being a parent if it is using your own eggs?
- Listen as your partner reassures you that they are with you because of

you. Believe them when they tell you they love you.

- Know that the uterus has some impact on the embryo. It cannot influence how a child looks, but it may influence the nature of the child.

Things that may be helpful

- Allowing some time to feel the distress and to work through whether using donor eggs could be okay for you.
- Believing your partner's reassurance.
- Talking to a few trusted friends or family members about your situation and letting them support you.
- Making a list of the things that help you—exercise, beaches, picnics, music and other things and people you enjoy—and attempting to do things on this list. (For ideas, see section entitled "Maintaining wellbeing – Resilience in times of waiting".)
- Using the counsellor at your clinic—they can help with your

feelings and give you a lot of information to help make decisions.

Chapter 15

Surrogacy

Surrogacy is a big event for two groups of parents—the hopeful intending parents and the surrogate woman or couple. Even in the most straightforward situations, from the time they approach the clinic for this treatment it may take nearly two years to get to completion. This covers the ethical application, treatment, pregnancy and birth and the three months postpartum for the surrogate, or as she is then known, the birth mother. It includes the interim adoption of the child by the intending parents but not the final adoption order.

Surrogacy involves having another woman carry a child for a couple or single person, heterosexual or gay, when they cannot have a pregnancy themselves. It allows them to become parents to a child who may have some genetic input from the intending parents. It is a long, sometimes complex journey that hopefully will provide remarkable joy for the new parents and a feeling of achievement and close connection to the new family for the surrogate family.

There are two groups who are the biggest users of surrogacy. Firstly, heterosexual couples where the woman is unable to carry a child for one of a variety of reasons. The second, and fastest-growing group, is male couples who, once adoption became available to them, have begun to use clinic-assisted surrogacy.

The potential to use surrogacy has been around for a very long time. The first written mention of surrogacy is in the Old Testament of the Bible when Abraham and Sarah asked their servant Hagar to carry a child for them. Traditional surrogacy, with the surrogate using her eggs and home inseminations, has long existed in the community. Clinics began, in the later 1970s, to experiment with traditional surrogacy, but it was not until 1985 that the first gestational surrogacy (using an egg that was not the surrogate's) was completed. The laws around surrogacy and adoption have been developed and refined since then and are still being actively worked upon.

When a woman carries a child for another person using her own egg inseminated with the sperm of the man who wishes to be parent, it is traditional surrogacy. With the development of IVF and fertilisation taking place in a laboratory, the capacity to use the potential mother's eggs or an egg donor's eggs became a possibility. As effective embryo freezing was developed, gestational surrogacy became a realistic possibility. In gestational surrogacy the surrogate carries a child who generally has no genetic link to her. Gestational surrogacy is the most frequent surrogacy to take place in the fertility clinic; infrequently traditional surrogacy may take place.

In New Zealand, surrogacy using a fertility clinic has a process through which all parties must proceed to be able to get treatment. It is guided by the HART Act 2004, which requires that each surrogacy situation must be approved by ECART. At the time of writing there are moves afoot to change some of the requirements of current ethical approval, such as having to adopt the child born from your genes. Law changes take some time.

The process for gestational surrogacy

When the fertility specialist confirms that surrogacy is the appropriate treatment for a couple, they begin on a pathway that at times will feel long and tedious, but which is designed to protect all participants and the surrogate's partner and children.

Ethical application

The ECART committee is a specialist group of professionals who meet about six times a year and receive applications from the fertility clinics to provide approval for surrogacy and other non-established treatments. The committee consists of members who represent a broad range of disciplines, professions and interests, including expertise in ethics, fertility, health and disability, Māori health and consumer advocacy. The guidelines and application forms used by the clinics are available for anyone to peruse on the web by putting 'ECART' into a search engine.

The process of getting the application ready to be sent to ECART and then considered, and receiving their response, can take about six months. Clinics cannot begin treatment until they have this approval—the making of embryos before there is a uterus to gestate them in is ethically not robust, so they must wait until ECART signals approval to begin.

The application the clinic sends to ECART will contain a medical report for each couple, individual couple counselling reports and a joint counselling report, and reports from the meetings with the lawyers who explain the legal ramifications. Oranga Tamariki has to approve IVF Surrogacy Adoption prior to the application going to ECART.

The ECART committee is required to look at the safety and wellbeing of all people involved in the application, including the intended child(ren). It looks to the HART Act for the founding principles. (See 'Appendix: the laws influencing fertility treatment'.)

For an application to be submitted by the fertility clinic to ECART, both of the intending parents, and the surrogate as well as a donor, if being used, will have:

- seen a fertility specialist for a medical assessment about suitability
- had two counselling sessions with a counsellor to look into the implications and decisions that surrogacy brings with it
- had a joint session between the intending parents and surrogate (and partner)
- had joint sessions with personally recruited donors
- received approval from Oranga Tamariki (intending parents)
- seen a lawyer familiar with the surrogacy and adoption laws.

The intending parents and surrogate need to have different medical specialists, counsellors and lawyers. Each of the doctors, counsellors and lawyers will complete the application forms for the ethics committee.

The fertility medical professionals look at the health of the surrogate, her previous pregnancies and births, the likely impact of a further birth, and her mental health. Under some circumstances they will refer the surrogate to an obstetric physician for specialist assessment. This occurs especially when a woman is older, heavier or has a medical condition or other health issues which create risk to her. It is important to recognise that what may be an appropriate risk for a woman to choose to take for her own pregnancy may not be an appropriate risk when she is carrying a child for someone else.

Medical consultation

When a couple comes to the clinic to explore surrogacy, they will first see the fertility specialist, who will decide whether surrogacy is the appropriate treatment. The specialist will look at the fertility health and general health of the couple, including any mental health issues. If relevant the specialist will seek other medical information. The reason for surrogacy will be discussed, including how the couple or person will access eggs and sperm. Any special tests that need to be done will be completed, and the specialist will inform them that counselling with a fertility counsellor is a mandatory part of this process. Often they know this and have made an appointment with the counsellor to follow the specialist consultation. The fertility specialist will use the information gathered from tests and the couple's information to write their medical report for ECART.

Role of Oranga Tamariki

In counselling, the couple or person will have time to discuss and understand the process of the ECART application, the treatment and hopefully a pregnancy through surrogacy. One of the first things the counsellor will suggest is that they begin the IVF Surrogacy Adoption approval process. Oranga Tamariki, the agency involved, need three to four months to approve the adoption, and this must be completed prior to submitting the ECART application. Once the child is born, the intending parent or parents will need to adopt the child so they become the guardian(s), and, with the final adoption order, the parent(s) on the birth certificate.

Counselling sessions

Counselling is the opportunity for the parties to consider the implications of the surrogacy. It ensures all parties are aware that the pregnancy will be very different from the surrogate's own pregnancies. It considers the impact on the surrogate of relinquishing the child to the intending parents following birth. Carrying a child which the surrogate will not parent is entirely different from carrying a child with the anticipation of parenting. It also affects the partner of the surrogate and their children. The partner and children will need to know how to respond to people's queries about their family's pregnancy, for example.

Each party (intending parents and surrogates) will have two individual counselling sessions, and sometimes they will need more. Counselling covers a multitude of subjects that help them understand the process of surrogacy.

One of the first discussion points often covers finding a surrogate. Some lucky people have a family member or friend who has offered to carry the pregnancy, but many have to seek a surrogate through their connections.

Once a surrogate has been found and agreed to proceed, each party, with their counsellor, will talk about optimum ways forward so they have a good surrogacy experience. The parties need to spend time talking to each other and learning about each other. This is often different knowledge from what we usually have about our friends, and is about understanding more intimate information about their lives—pregnancies, births and how the intending parents might fit into this.

The surrogate and her partner become the original birth parents for the child. They will have a lifetime connection and the child will need to know of their beginnings, so building an early relationship and having a clear understanding of the values and expectations of each party is fundamental to the success of this long process. Both parties need to be able to trust the process. The surrogate needs to feel sure the intending parents will support her in pregnancy and will adopt the child following birth. The intending parents have to trust that the surrogate will care for the baby in pregnancy and relinquish the baby after birth.

The parties are often shocked when told they need to allow about two years for the whole surrogacy process. The surrogate family need to think about, and try to anticipate, where their family will be in two years and how this might fit into their lives. The hopeful parents will be planning and getting ready for the child while feeling a bit out of control as they watch their pregnancy develop from a distance.

Counselling also involves the intending parents developing an understanding of pregnancy and how this pregnancy is likely to affect the surrogate. They need to think about the support they can offer the surrogate family, and to realise that the support needed at the beginning is very different from that needed at the end of the pregnancy. The HART Act is very clear: payment or valuable consideration for the surrogacy is illegal. Surrogacy is altruistic, with only pregnancy-related expenses being able to be paid for by the intending parents. Most intending parents support the surrogate and her family by very practical means, such as providing childcare over weekends, cooking meals for the freezer and other things they can provide practically. Surrogates seldom want more than interest and friendship during the first two trimesters, but as the foetus becomes bigger and the pregnancy harder they are happy to have support of a practical nature. Most surrogates find it hard to ask for support, so the intending parents need to be open and forward about checking on needs. Communication is important here so the support can change and increase as needed.

Counselling will also look at the role of the intending parents in the birth experience. It will help the two parties develop a plan for the relinquishment of the child and understand the legal processes that are needed at that time.

In both individual and joint counselling the issue of termination will be discussed until all parties feel they have an agreed stance on this. Most will find it realistic and acceptable that any risk to the birth mother (surrogate) will involve a termination, but they find it harder to consider abnormality in the child as a reason for terminating this much-wanted pregnancy. Ultimately the birth mother has the final say and signs the papers for a termination, but few birth mothers wish it to be their decision alone; they want to feel supported and have everyone in agreement with the decision. Some of the situations that parties have had to contemplate include Downs syndrome or more generally situations where the quality of life for the child will be low if it survives birth. There are many different ways the foetus can have problems, and the general principles for making a decision need to be considered. Fortunately having talked their way through this issue most of the parties do not have to face this reality.

They will also discuss how they will react if a child is born with an abnormality—whether there is any chance the child could be rejected by the intending parents and what would happen then. Both parties need to feel clear about the guardianship plans for the child if anything happens to any participant in pregnancy.

Legal aspects and lawyer consultations

Each party has to see an independent lawyer to have the legal aspects of the treatment and adoption explained. The lawyer will inform them of the laws relevant to the surrogacy situation and explain how they are relevant. They will help each party understand the legal issues, such as their rights during the pregnancy and following birth, the adoption process and payment of expenses. This will be covered in their report for ECART. The lawyer will also help them understand the steps they need to take for the adoption as they get towards the end of the pregnancy and the birth of the child. The intending parents need to understand that until the interim adoption order (at 10 working days after birth) is through, they have no legal rights to the child. They need to understand the costs around adoption and be able to plan for this.

The surrogate also needs to be fully informed about her role in the process of adoption and the requirements of her and her partner. Her lawyer will ensure she has this information.

Next steps

Once ECART approval is given, the next stage can proceed. If there are embryos in the freezer the surrogate can use them; if not, there is an IVF cycle to create embryos that then need to be frozen for three months to exclude issues of infection.

Achieving a pregnancy is the next step, and it may take more than one attempt with a frozen embryo to get a viable pregnancy. Once pregnant, there are the nine months of pregnancy before birth. This pregnancy may be very different and often somewhat harder than the surrogate's previous pregnancies. The postpartum period of three months is important, as in this time the surrogate is working through the emotions of relinquishing the child and of her body and family returning to normal. The new parents are learning to cope with the baby and are working through the adoption process.

Isobel and Mike

Isobel and Mike were aware they would need surrogacy as Isobel was born without a uterus. They learned what they could about the surrogacy process, then began to look for a surrogate. Having ruled out close family—neither had sisters—they set about letting friends know in the hope they might find someone. While they were waiting and hoping, Mike's brother and his wife came to offer to be their surrogate parents. Johnny and Sheila had finished their family, and they felt they could do this with the support of all the family.

This wonderful offer took Isobel and Mike by surprise, and they suggested Johnny and Sheila talk with the fertility specialist and counsellor at the clinic to hear about the implications and check whether Sheila would be able to safely have a fourth pregnancy.

This began the process of five months for the ECART application to be approved, then two months while Isobel and Mike had IVF and made embryos. There was a quarantine period before Sheila had the embryo placed into her uterus, and they were lucky with the second embryo to get a confirmation of pregnancy.

The pregnancy was—as they were warned pregnancies without a genetic link to the surrogate are likely to be—much more difficult than Sheila's own pregnancies, but finally at 39 weeks the child was born. They signed the interim adoption papers 12 days later.

Sheila and Johnny felt great that they had achieved their goal in giving Mike and Isobel a child to parent. They also recognised how challenging the whole process had been for them and their children, and they were glad to settle back into their normal life. The child, born 23 months after they first talked with Isobel and Mike, would always be special to them. It is the joy on Isobel and Mike's faces that Sheila and Johnny recall when they think about the experience.

Involvement of gamete or embryo donors

Surrogacy can happen in a number of ways when a donor is involved—either a sperm donor or an egg donor. It is possible to use both egg and sperm donors or an embryo donor with surrogacy. Whether people use a personally recruited donor or a clinic-recruited donor, the donor needs to understand that the intending mother will not carry the pregnancy and decide if they feel comfortable with the use of a surrogate. Sometimes the donors may wish to meet the surrogate parents. This is not required by ECART.

The donors will have counselling, and reports will be written for ECART outlining their understanding of the process, the relationship to the intending parents, and the knowledge that the child will need to have access to her/his genetic information in the future.

Male couples and surrogacy

While some of the aspects of surrogacy are particular to male couples, much is the same as for heterosexual couples. This chapter is relevant to both. 'Chapter 11: Same-gender relationships' covers the information about surrogacy that is specific to men.

Danny and Kyle

Danny and Kyle have been together 10 years. They married two years ago but only recently decided to look into having children. Danny is the driver for this and so he did the ground work, reading about surrogacy in New Zealand and looking at blogs about other men who had successfully had children in this country.

He quickly ascertained there were a number of pitfalls if they did a DIY with a woman found on a website. The most worrying was the lack of legal right they had to the child. The men rang the clinic and asked for someone to talk with. The receptionist suggested they make an appointment with the counsellor who could give them the required information.

The men wrote a list of questions they wanted answered about their rights to the child and about their roles as well as those of the donor and the surrogate following birth. The counsellor began by telling them the processes they would need to undertake—adoption approval with Oranga Tamariki, application to ECART, IVF cycle for the donor, quarantine of embryos and replacing the embryos into the surrogate. It sounded like such a lot of work, but as the counsellor pointed out, this is done over a period of time—it's a step-by-step process. They also briefly talked about the men needing to understand pregnancy and childbirth in order to support their surrogate.

The counsellor then worked through their questions until the men felt they had enough information to take home and consider the next steps.

Thinking ahead—the pregnancy and birth

Becoming pregnant is exciting at the best of times, and especially when there are two couples involved, and potentially a donor. The level of excitement is high. Through the clinic people hear about their pregnancy at four weeks gestation. This is a time when there is a risk of miscarriage. Most miscarriages occur when the embryo (which in early stages drives the pregnancy) is not able to take the pregnancy further. Once a heartbeat is established the risk drops a bit, but it is when the placenta takes over maintaining the pregnancy that it becomes relatively safe. It is commonly thought the pregnancy is relatively safe if all is well at the ultrasound scan at 13 weeks.

Because the surrogate is carrying an embryo that is genetically unlinked to her she may have more nausea and fatigue in her first trimester than she did with her own children. Hopefully this will diminish at the beginning of the second trimester, but if it is too hard she needs to seek medical advice. The intending parents can be helpful, if the surrogate is happy for them to do so, by providing some meals that just need heating, helping with her children and just generally being available if she and her partner need support.

The second trimester is more likely to be an easier one for the surrogate and family. It is as she enters the third trimester and begins to have a large tummy and feel heavy that she may struggle with the family tasks and appreciate extra support from the intending parents. Because most intending parents have no experience of pregnancy they are wise to ask what support would be useful rather than try to assume they will get it right. Practical support is always a good place to start—helping with her children and their activities, or if she is a single woman doing her garden and lawns. There are many tasks that allow the intending parents to feel they are contributing to the surrogate's wellbeing without contravening the valuable consideration aspect of the HART Act.

Planning for the birth and the roles of each person is particular to each situation. Some surrogates want their intending parents in the room and fully involved during birth, others want them at the 'head end' only, and yet others want them to come into the room following birth. These things can be worked out over time. Ultimately the goal is having a healthy baby, a well surrogate and all parties feeling as if they have done the best they are able to do.

Following birth

After birth the baby can be with the intending parents providing they and their surrogate have sorted this out with Oranga Tamariki before the birth.

The surrogate, or birth mother as she is generally called, then enters the 'fourth trimester' of pregnancy. She has had a child but does not have a baby at home, and while she will not want the child at home she may need to see the child for reassurance over the next while. She is likely to want to introduce the child to her children, who have been aware of the pregnancy and would love to meet the baby and have a cuddle, then acknowledge it lives in another family. The birth family would probably like a photograph of the child, so as the time-distance gets greater they can reflect on the photo and a task well done.

The birth mother's body will take a while to return to pre-pregnancy state and her emotions will settle over time. This is a challenging time for the birth mother and her family as they move back to life within their family unit.

The new family will also be trying to come to terms with their lives being changed dramatically by this longed-for little person who now rules their family.

Janet

Janet was a surrogate for her beloved sister and her sister's partner, and gave them the child they longed for but could not produce themselves. As she was warned, it was a tough pregnancy. She sought support from both her midwife and counsellor regularly to help her deal with it.

Janet had a lot more pregnancy symptoms and often felt nauseous and unable to work for longer than with her own pregnancies. She always said she did not love being pregnant but loved the end product.

Possibly her biggest challenge came as a result of her openness about the surrogacy. It became the only thing people talked to her about, and she found she was feeling lost as a person. With the counsellor's support she began a campaign to gently say to all those who raised the issue that she was having time off talking about the surrogacy, and then she asked what was happening in their life. This worked a treat.

Janet's intending parents were amazing, they helped with her children, provided meals, took over the housework and made it possible for Janet and her partner to continue with their work routines.

Following the birth Janet commented that she knew she had done a very special thing for her sister and she was glad she had had the opportunity. She was surprised by how tricky the pregnancy had been emotionally, and how at times it had felt very long. She had no regrets, but was very glad to put back together the pieces of her and her family's life.

Things to think about

- What are you looking for in a surrogate? Does she need to have finished her family? Can she live overseas? When is too old? If she has had C sections, does that rule her out? What health issues rule her out? How well do you need to know her?
- How will you feel having a surrogate carry your child?

- What relationship will you want with her and her family after the surrogacy is over?
- Have you thought about how to support the surrogate family and checked with them that this is acceptable to them?

Things that might be helpful

- Reading and understanding as much as you can before starting the process.
- Ensuring the specialist at the clinic believes this is the appropriate treatment for you before getting too involved.
- While it is hard to find a surrogate, be sure to consider (before you ask her) having this person in your life, and that of your child, forever.
- For both parties, recognise that the process (ECART, treatment, pregnancy and post-birth) generally takes about two years—this is a long time to be consumed by the process before you move to the next stage of life.

- If your surrogate is a bit needy in pregnancy and you feel she is asking a lot of you, recognise that she cannot get away from your pregnancy. Take a deep breath and talk about how to manage this stage. Or all go to counselling and have a sort-out.
- Often it is a smart idea to have a joint counselling session at about 25 weeks of pregnancy to plan for the final stages.

Chapter 16

Secondary infertility

Secondary infertility occurs when a woman has a child or children and is unable to become pregnant again. The woman may have conceived readily previously and carried the child without difficulty and as a result she may not acknowledge there is a problem for some time. She may feel a strong sense of disbelief that there could be a problem. Yet secondary infertility is as common as primary infertility, it is just less well known. Those who struggle with secondary infertility report there is little sympathy for those who have it. They are often told to enjoy the child they have without people recognising that few of us want to settle for one child.

Most people, when they begin their journey to become parents, will have some idea of the number of children they ideally would like to have. Commonly this reflects the family size they grew up within their family of origin. In New Zealand the average woman's age for the birth of the first child is 31, and the average New Zealand family has 1.9 children per household. These figures have been fairly stable over the past decade.

Rebecca and Sean

Rebecca and Sean had several years together before they had their first child. Rebecca wanted to have her first child when she was around 30 years old, and they were both 30 when they stopped the contraceptive pill. They conceived after about four months of trying for a child, and their son was born without complications. Both Rebecca and Sean were the oldest in families with two children, and they also planned to have a second child.

When their son was 18 months old they stopped contraception and hoped they would conceive relatively quickly so the children were close and likely to engage in the same activities. By the time their son was four years old they were ready to admit they needed help. At this stage both Rebecca and Sean were 35 years old, so still within the range of ages where they should be able to conceive.

When the couple came to their clinic consultation they had both done a number of tests, none of which gave any indication of the reason they were not conceiving. The doctor talked with them about giving Rebecca's ovulation a small boost with stimulant drugs while they did some more advanced tests. The couple then went to see the nurse for further information. The nurse recognised they were fragile, both individually and as a couple, and suggested they talk with the counsellor about strategies for coping with what might be a long haul.

A few days later Rebecca and Sean came to talk with the counsellor, and as Sean said it was a great relief to be able to talk of their fears and the impact it was having on them. They had been getting into blaming and arguing. They said their biggest issue was their son wanting a sibling and their sadness about the size of the age gap. Rebecca felt under pressure as she watched her coffee-group friends have second children and return to work, and she felt they were losing this group of friends. She had worked hard to get Sean to seek help.

The couple seemed bleak. They expressed concern about this issue not being able to be resolved. They were not eligible for funded treatment and could not afford an IVF cycle. They had agreed they would have three months of attempts with this low-level treatment and then stop treatment all together.

Discussion centred around managing grief, both as it was now and as Rebecca had her periods each month. We talked about ways for them to support each other and things they might do to strengthen their relationship.

Their worst-case scenario of being a family of three was raised and acknowledged as not their ideal. Some alternative ways of looking at this and giving their son companionship were discussed. These ideas were acknowledged early so if their current treatment was not successful they could see something of life after treatment.

PS: Rebecca and Sean were not successful in their desire to have another child using ovulation induction. They were aware that in two years they would be eligible to go on the list for a government-funded cycle with about an 18-month wait on the list before they could have treatment. They decided they would settle for being a family of three people and take the opportunities this presented. At the time of this meeting they were beginning to grasp life again and feel as if they were going to enjoy their future together.

For this couple no reason could be found for their secondary infertility. For other people the cause of secondary infertility may be similar reasons to primary infertility—male factors, female factors or combined issues. For a number of women age can be a factor in secondary infertility. As a woman's age increases it causes a decline in her fertility with some variation about when that decline begins. The wait after the birth of the first child in the hope of a natural conception may mean her age is no longer ideal.

Typically, a couple will try for quite a long time for their subsequent child, not recognising they may need help to conceive. Each month brings a cycle of hope as they are sure they were making love over the fertile time, then anxiety as they wait for the bleeding in the menstrual cycle. They will watch their friends have child number two and sometimes number three before they acknowledge they are not succeeding by themselves and it may be time to seek help. During the time of trying, their lives and relationships are likely to be affected by the pressure to provide a sibling for their child. This can impact on their relationship and intimacy, changing the focus from the pleasure in being together to the task of trying to conceive. Inevitably as time for a period arrives, the anxiety creeps up and the couple may find themselves at odds or tiptoeing around each other. This is very stressful for both people.

As time goes on friends and family feel it is acceptable to ask when they intend to have another child, and the couple often find a lot of excuses to maintain their privacy. Being asked about a subsequent child emphasises their lack of success and often results in their avoiding some people. If the couple have several people asking, they will often feel quite isolated. Sometimes family or friends say they should be glad they at least have the child(ren) they have. This may make the couple feel guilty about wanting another child. They are glad they have a child, they just want what others have—another child. One of the biggest differences between primary infertility and secondary infertility is that these people know what they are missing out on—pregnancy and another child to love. This poses a significant grief for them.

As their child goes to preschool they will see other children get a sibling and might innocently ask if they are going to get one also. This adds to the parents' grief, and they may be unsure how to respond to this question. When their child asks this question, parents need to keep in mind the child is asking a question about something they have observed. Their child only understands having both parents to themselves and not how life changes when you have a sibling in the family. The parents' yearning can be transferred to the child, and sometimes when the child recognises this is a place to get parental reaction they will talk about it frequently.

It is up to the parents of this only child to ensure their quest for another child does not become the child's search also. The child needs to know their parents enjoy the family as it is and that they love being their parent. If the child is taught there is a gap in the family they wonder if it is them, the child, not being quite enough.

Occasionally a mother will 'confess' her child is her best friend and confidant. This upsets the balance in a family as it involves the child taking care of the parent at an age when they should be learning about life and friendships with children. The making of babies is the business of parents and should not be of concern to the child. Parents often acknowledge to the child that they would like to have another child but they may not be able to have one, but they should keep the emotions around this to themselves so the child is not burdened by them and feel they have a role in this. Children will accept the inform ation when it is told as another of the bits of knowledge that belongs to their family.

The public funding as it is allocated now means that clinics often create families with one child. This is not the ideal many hoped for at the beginning of their treatment lives.

Using donor gametes to have another child

Sometimes the biological clock has run too far for a child to be born using the couple's own gametes, and for the couple to have another child there will need to be a donor involved. While this is more commonly an egg donor because the woman is moving into early menopause, there are times when the man's sperm is no longer viable. Either of these situations is distressing to the couple, particularly as it is a change they will not have been aware of and they may not know the cause of this change.

As with all people who find they need donor gametes, there is grief to be worked through before this option is used. (See 'Chapter 13: Donor sperm' and 'Chapter 14: Donor eggs'.)

Having a child who is genetically connected to both parents and then having a donor child needs to be considered carefully. The donor will bring a different genetic input to the child, and the parents need to think through how they will manage this in the future. They will need to consider such issues as how they will find a donor and what they hope to find in this donor. They need to think about the story they will tell the child of their conception and genetic origins—children are often very aware of themselves as different within a family, and their identity is best formed when they have the correct information and are able to integrate it into the knowledge they have of themselves. Parents need to think about behaving in a way that both children feel loved and equally enjoyed for their own traits. Most people know that any two children in a family will be different. This will be true in this family also.

Advantages of a single-child family

There are known advantages to children growing up as the only child in a family. While there are some aspects of family life they will not experience, there are other things they will gain from. It is very difficult for people desperately wanting a further child to see that there are advantages in a family with one child. Yet a number of the people who try to add another child to their family will, for a variety of reasons, remain a family of three people. These reasons may include the cost of treatment being beyond them and no government funding available, the only treatment available being using a donor and the couple do not wish to do this, that treatment is unsuccessful, or that they just feel they cannot cope with the pressure treatment brings to them.

Some couples will recognise the benefits of a small family and work out the advantages they feel. For some there is a cousin who is a favourite of their child, so the children spend lots of time together. Others ensure their child interacts with other children frequently. Most smaller families encourage the child to become self-contained in play for periods of each day. This capacity to entertain themselves is a useful skill for young people in their future.

Children who grow up as only children tend to be socially competent and able to accommodate others who bring difference. With the blend of time spent socialising and time alone they learn to cope with situations and become stable as adults. The input they have from their two parents has significant benefits for them—plenty of attention, support and access to resources. Most of the parents of single children can afford to involve the child in activities where they can socialise with other children. The parents do not have to share their time between several children, so they interact with their child more frequently. They are there to help them process the world and to develop independence. These are useful skills to take into the world, which requires both competent relationships but also independence.

Callum and Katrina

Callum and Katrina became pregnant with Lucy easily not long after they got together. Katrina loved being pregnant, and many of her fantasies were based around at least one further experience of this.

When they had not conceived a second time after two years of trying, they wanted help and the doctor at the clinic told them they were unlikely to conceive again as Katrina had a very low ovarian reserve. If they used donor eggs, they would be likely to have another child.

Callum was happy to settle for one child, but Katrina became very down and eventually sought help from her GP. As well as prescribing some medication, the GP referred her to community-based counselling. She worked hard on her depression and began to regain her sense of what was important for them. She had to learn to rethink her internal fantasies. She also looked at the reality of the cost for an egg-donor cycle, and together she and Callum decided not to proceed with it.

Katrina retrained in a new career once Lucy was in school. She says she still has times of sadness but is busy making sure their lives are full and happy.

In a small family resources do not have to be spread as far and so these children tend to be more educated and to have their parents involved in their education. While not learning to share the resources, including attention, can be a disadvantage, all children have the great leveller of school where they cannot be the only shining star and have to share the limelight.

There are both positive and negative aspects to all family sizes, and for the adults it is important to recognise and work through the grief that you cannot have your ideal size easily. Following this the couple need to look at options and ensure that they make the family size they have work well for them and their child.

Things to think about

- What do you enjoy about your family as it is?
- How can you look after each other as you go through this experience?
- What impact is this having on your relationship?
- Do you both want this subsequent child equally?
- Can you talk about this without arguments, or should you find someone to support you in your talking?
- Should you get to the doctor earlier, at least to exclude issues?
- Constantly review how far you will go to have subsequent children.

Things that might be helpful

- Finding someone you trust to talk with about how this affects you. This will reduce the isolation and help you process the information about the implications.
- Taking time as a couple to share this fear. Listening to your partner, and not interrupting while they process their feelings, is very important. Feeling heard makes a person feel valued.
- Understanding that your partner's feelings may change over time, and accepting that. We cannot tell others how they should feel.
- Acknowledging to each other that while you are grateful and lucky to have your child, you would love to have another. You do not have to justify this, it is enough to yearn to have another.
- Ensuring you do things together that you enjoy and also maintaining the family activities that work for you all.
- Working out what it is you want to say if you agree to share this

information with close people. It is okay to tell them and minimise discussion about it.

Chapter 17

Age-related infertility

Our society has changed, and this is reflected in the lives of all of us and especially women. Women may seek more education, a career, they may wish to travel, pay off student loans, or become financially stable before they consider having children. Sometimes women may take longer to settle in a relationship, and consequently are older when they try to conceive. The one thing that stays the same is the distress that occurs as they fail to get pregnant.

New Zealanders have the belief that if you work hard at something and set up optimum conditions then you will get a positive result. Fertility does not always fit with this belief. As people age, their eggs and sperm age also, and while taking care of yourself is good it will not bring back young eggs or sperm.

There are some lucky people who do have children when one or both parties are older. Having tests will help decide how likely this might be, and help plan how to proceed from there. Current treatments may enhance the possibility. In New Zealand there is no government funding for people when a woman is over 40 years—the Ministry of Health believe that putting the scarce fertility money where they believe it is most likely to be successful is the best plan.

Some women use donated eggs to achieve a family when they hear they are unlikely to conceive any other way. There are many issues to consider before making this decision and reading the chapter about using a donor ('Chapter 12: Using a donor—eggs and sperm') and the one about donor eggs ('Chapter 14: Donor eggs') will give you some insight into these issues.

'I have never been this fit and healthy in my life, yet I cannot get pregnant.' (Jessie, aged 41)

'My mother had her third child at 43, I should be able to be like her.' (Adele, aged 42)

Sentiments similar to the above are often heard by counsellors. They are cries of disbelief and distress. They indicate the woman either does not know about the impact of age on her fertility or does not want to acknowledge that this information applies to her.

The distress at not conceiving takes time to work through. Initially the woman (or couple) may look around and see others within a few years of her age who are having children or they might read in magazines about stars who conceive even in their late forties (without an acknowledgement they are using donated eggs). If others can do it they feel they too should be able to conceive. But each woman is an individual and will have a different fertility status, so comparisons with friends or family—or strangers—may not be valid.

Managing distress can take a lot of forms. Firstly, becoming informed about the impact of age helps with the cognitive recognition about your lack of conception. Emotionally you will need to recognise that you are likely to have a well of sadness about not becoming parents, and this infiltrates your lives. This is accentuated by many of the day-to-day things that focus on families with children. You may find it difficult to visit friends with children, and especially those who have new babies. You may not want to be best aunty and uncle at birthday parties, and public holidays such as Christmas may become very difficult for you.

In recognising and acknowledging you have a fertility problem, you give yourselves options to behave differently. Some people may be able to tell their friends they are having difficulty getting pregnant, but many feel this is a private area of their lives. Once the secret is shared though, friends and family will understand if a couple behaves differently. For example, when a new baby is born the couple can visit their friends and the new child once they are at home rather than in the birthing unit. This means they are less confronted by the world of new babies and others' successes.

Laura and Richard

LAURA: Finally at 39 I decided we needed to get onto it. Deep down I think I knew it might not happen. I became super-aware of all the babies and pregnancies around me, and increasingly they made me upset. I knew I was becoming hell to live with. Richard suggested I find someone to talk with, so I went to talk with the counsellor at the clinic. We worked out that I could make some changes that made sure we still had a life—doing things we knew were good for us. When I wept while talking about all the friends' pregnancies and children, she asked why I was focusing on those particular friends. I was stunned and knew she was right. Because I wanted to be in that situation it was like I hoped fertility might be contagious. So I identified those of our friends who were past that stage and resolved to spend more time with them. I made a decision in this discussion that I would acknowledge baby showers with a wee gift but not attend, and would visit a new baby when it was a bit older than newborn.

Richard and I also decided that evening that we would not spend the coming Christmas with our large extended families but would go away and have adventures together. We emailed our families to tell them, including the reasons, and they all supported us.

These practical ideas helped us feel more in control.

One of the costs of telling people is that they will want to understand and help. Sometimes this talking is welcome, other times not. Some support comes in the form of stories and advice, neither of which are easy to listen to. Sometimes it helps to take away the isolation, other times it is hard to hear. A handy tool for this situation is to gently say, 'I would rather not talk about this now.'

For the couple, or single woman, it is important to ensure your life is still moving along with the areas of success that you know and experience. Activities such as work, exercise, social activities and community activities all support you while you get through these difficult times. Lack of success in becoming pregnant does not invalidate all the fields in which you are successful. Nobody is just one area of life, even when it is such an important area. The disappointment and sadness does need to be managed so as not to become all-consuming.

Gathering information to understand what and why this is happening, including doing tests that will look at your specific situation, helps to deal with distress and with moving forward to look for a solution.

Statistics

The clinics all produce informative and easy-to-read websites and booklets so you can feel well informed. To put this chapter into context: conception rates for normal healthy couples under 35 are usually around 20–25 per cent per menstrual cycle. Once you reach the age of 35, your fertility begins to decline. By age 40, it is estimated that your conception rate is in the range of 8–10 per cent per month, and at age

43 the pregnancy rate is thought to be as low as 1–3 per cent per month. By age 45, fertility has declined so much that getting pregnant naturally is unlikely for most women.

Women are born with all the eggs they will ever have, and by puberty the number will have dropped from a few million to around 300,000. By menopause it is less than 1000. For each egg that matures and is released each menstrual cycle, there are some that do not mature and are absorbed back into your body.

As the number decreases so does the quality, although this is not well understood. As you age, the chromosomal material in the eggs also ages, making them less capable of being fertilised or of continuing a pregnancy.

Miscarriage rates double for women between 35 and 45 from 25 per cent to 50 per cent. The chance of Downs syndrome at 35 years is 1 in 170; at 45 years it is 1 in 11.

About 10 per cent of women experience menopause five years earlier than the average, and a small number 10 years earlier.

Toni and Jeremy

Toni and Jeremy came to the clinic as a 41-year-old woman and 50-year-old man. They had met a few years earlier and decided they wanted a child in their lives. They had friends who had had successful IVF, and when they did not conceive naturally they had a strong sense that IVF was the pathway for them also.

Prior to seeing the specialist they were asked to do a series of blood tests and, for Jeremy, a semen analysis. Toni had an FSH and an AMH. FSH (follicle-stimulating hormone) tells the doctor how hard the pituitary gland has to work to stimulate production of an egg, and AMH (anti-mullerian hormone) indicates the reserve number of eggs in the ovaries.

The specialist gave them the sad information that Toni's FSH was high, indicating the pituitary gland had to work very hard and was probably unable to stimulate eggs, and her AMH was at 1, telling them she had few eggs in her ovaries. Toni was devastated, having believed IVF could solve their problems and now hearing this was unlikely.

The couple made an appointment with the doctor's nurse a couple of days later to get her to go over the information the doctor had given them, as once they heard the bad news they thought they might have stopped listening. The nurse confirmed what they had heard, and gently introduced the idea of using donor eggs so they could be parents. Toni and Jeremy felt completely unready for this, so she suggested they go on a fact-finding mission and talk to the counsellor about it. She gave them an information brochure on donor eggs for when they were ready.

It took some time before they were able to own the fact that they needed to at least get the information so they could make an informed decision. During this time they had begun to share their news with family so they could receive the support they needed.

In counselling they learned about the implications of using donor eggs, thinking firstly about themselves and their child, then about the donor and her children. They talked about obtaining a donor and how embryos were made from the donor eggs. As important, they got some strategies for dealing with the distress of not being able to have a fully genetic child, and again they went away to digest this information.

Sometime later they reappeared with Toni's younger cousin Jess, aged 33, who wanted to learn about what it took to donate eggs.

Their child was born when Toni was 43, and had some of her genes through the cousin relationship with Jess. The baby gave great pleasure to all the family, who had felt so unsure of how to help Toni and Jeremy. With all the family knowing of the donation, Jess was well supported and appreciated through the IVF. Toni and Jeremy and their treasured child acknowledged how lucky they were to have this opportunity and then be successful.

Men and aging

While the age of men has an impact on their fertility, it is different from women and may not be as significant in conception. Men, as they age, are likely to have fewer sperm, and their quality, like women's eggs, will be affected by age. It seems to happen more gradually in men and may not impact on their ability, through IVF, to fertilise a younger egg. In IVF, sperm selection can happen through ICSI (intracytoplasmic sperm injection) when one sperm is injected into each egg. This is helpful when numbers are too low to fertilise an egg naturally.

As men move up through their late forties they need to be aware there are implications for the chromosomal material in their sperm, with issues beginning after about 45. Overseas studies indicate older sperm may raise the level of risk for a child having autism or schizophrenia.

Parenting at an older age

Whether or not people are lucky enough to have a child using their own or donor eggs when they are into their forties, the families created often have only one child. These children are much-loved and given lots of opportunities in life. They usually have parents who have a lot of life experience and are fairly settled, stable as a couple and financially secure.

Things to think about

- How far are you prepared to go to have a child? Many treatments? Significant cost?
- Would you consider using a donor?
- Having read the chapters on donations, would you still consider a donor?
- What would life be like without children? (See Chapter 20.)
- Where is the 'line in the sand' when you have done enough?

- Do you both want children equally? Talk about this if you have very different ideas.
- What might make your relationship at risk?

Things that might be helpful

- Writing a list of all the things that are important in your life. Are you still doing these things, or has your life narrowed as you seek a child?
- Looking at your friends and family and recognising the stages of life they are in. Does this indicate who might be able to be most supportive of you, either in helping you keep a life balance or in your quest for children?
- Making sure you are as healthy as possible.
- Becoming informed so you can understand the information at the clinic.
- Recognising there is life without a child if you need to do this.

Chapter 18

Pregnancy loss

Having fertility issues is difficult and needing treatment challenging. For a small group of those who have treatment the challenge increases when, having finally achieved the longed-for pregnancy, there is a pregnancy loss. The grief, sadness and sense of failure felt with fertility issues are all compounded with a pregnancy loss.

Following fertility treatment, a pregnancy is confirmed at the equivalent of four weeks of pregnancy. Usually a repeat test is done about four days later to confirm that the levels of hCG, the pregnancy hormone, are rising appropriately for an ongoing pregnancy. Mostly these levels rise normally, but sometimes at these blood tests there are indications that the pregnancy is unlikely to be ongoing. Hearing this news causes distress, but until the woman has signs of bleeding she will have a certain amount of disbelief and hope. Infrequently in these cases the pregnancy will proceed normally, but most often the hormones do not continue to rise at the required level as the routine weekly blood tests are undertaken.

Blood tests are usually done until an ultrasound scan can be done at around seven weeks to look at the size of the embryo and look for a heartbeat. Most pregnancy losses occur before this time, or the scan indicates that things are not proceeding as needed and the loss will happen soon.

Kimberly

Kimberly had used donor sperm and had a positive pregnancy test after her second round of IUI. She was thrilled with the news. She asked about the levels of hCG and the nurses told her that they were still rising as expected and to be hopeful. They also talked with her about the signs to watch out for with pregnancy loss or ectopic pregnancy.

All seemed to proceed normally and she took her mum to the seven-week scan. She was very glad of the support. She saw the baby's heartbeat and it was explained the baby had a slow heart rate. This slowness was not a good sign. She was to stay on drugs to support the pregnancy and have another scan in a week.

Kimberly went home feeling as if she was in limbo. On one level her blood tests were all fine and she had no bleeding or pain. Her breasts were tender and she had a full feeling in her tummy. These were the things she associated with pregnancy. When she allowed other thoughts to intrude, she felt deep sadness and she was aware the nurses had indicated she needed to be prepared for the loss of this pregnancy.

Her mother again came to the next scan. They saw immediately that there was no heartbeat. The baby had died and she would now have a miscarriage. The sadness and unfairness of the situation overwhelmed Kimberly. *Why me? Why can other people have babies that they don't even want? What did I do wrong that caused this?*

By chance the counsellor had a little time and sat with Kimberly and her mother while Kimberly wept and talked about her feelings. Kimberly was not ready to process the event straight after learning about the pregnancy loss, so the counsellor sorted out a time when they could have a talk and think about how she could go forward.

Pregnancy loss happens in about one in five pregnancies, usually in the early stages of the pregnancy. It occurs at the same rate in people who have had fertility treatment as it does in those who have conceived naturally. Early in pregnancy, genetic issues are a major cause of miscarriage, and these generally cause the embryo to stop growing at an early stage. It is commonly thought this may be nature's way of ensuring if the baby has problems it does not continue to grow. Of course this is not actually known, as few pregnancy-loss embryos are tested to see if they are normal. Usually a woman has to have more than three pregnancy losses before testing of the products from the pregnancy occurs.

Many women have a miscarriage at some stage, and only a few have more than one. The rate of miscarriage is more frequent as women grow older. There is very little either the woman or the health professionals can do to prevent or stop a pregnancy loss. Taking care of yourself both physically and emotionally are the most important things when a miscarriage is occurring and for the period afterwards.

Physical indications of a miscarriage

In some instances there may not be any signs the pregnancy is not flourishing. The support drugs given in treatment may prevent bleeding, but some women's bodies just continue to grow the placental sac even when the embryo has stopped growing.

Women who have some bleeding will generally call the nurses at their clinic. They are likely to be asked how much bleeding there is as an early assessment. They may be told that many women have a little bleeding and then go on to have successful pregnancies. It will be suggested they do another blood test to see if their hCG levels are still appropriate. They may also be told to rest quietly for a little time to see if the bleeding stops. If the bleeding is heavy the nurse will suggest they do another blood test, but she will also help them prepare for the likelihood of miscarriage.

Bleeding, pain similar to period cramps and a loss of the early symptoms of pregnancy such as tender breasts, fatigue or nausea are the common indicators women will feel at this early stage. Once bleeding becomes established it will be similar to a heavy period and will often have a number of blood clots. Sometimes these symptoms will be frightening for the woman and she may need her partner, mother or a friend as support. If the pain is too great she will need to go to A&E to make sure the pregnancy loss is happening normally. With a lot of pain the pregnancy might be ectopic, and in this instance the woman will need hospital care.

In most instances the woman will pass the tissues that formed the baby and the placenta naturally herself. Sometimes she will not pass them or may not pass all of them. This may require a D&C, a small procedure done under anaesthetic to remove the tissues of the pregnancy.

Emotional impact of pregnancy loss

When the phone call from the nurse confirms you are pregnant, your hopes are fulfilled. An excitement begins and quickly the early pregnancy becomes a child. The dreams and fantasies about life with a child and becoming parents begin. These dreams quickly turn into expectations of life going forward, so the loss of your pregnancy is shattering. It is the loss of hopes, dreams and expectations for the future. All these wonderful dreams have to be given up for now.

The physical loss of your pregnancy is not pleasant, and feeling sorrow and a sense of being cheated is normal. Sometimes you may feel guilt about the loss, shame about not being able to carry a pregnancy further and anger at everything because this is happening to you. These are common feelings. Occasionally you may have trouble sleeping, loss of appetite, irritability and an inability to focus on anything else, particularly in the early stages.

These emotions of sadness, anger, guilt and shame are all part of the grief that it is necessary to get through with this experience. Some people are able to do this more easily and quickly by using their cognitive skills to rationalise the event. They may say to themselves and others that nature was ensuring they did not have a baby with problems. They also may say the pregnancy did not feel strong from the beginning so they were not surprised. Some are able to say, well, I got past the hurdle of getting pregnant, now next time I want to stay pregnant.

For others the grief at needing fertility treatment is compounded by the miscarriage and becomes a significant hurdle to overcome. Being childless and having a miscarriage can seem like losing the last chance at being a parent. While most people are able to reconcile this within a year, some may need to talk with their family doctor or seek counselling to deal with depression.

Men and women both grieve when pregnancy loss occurs, but they tend to mourn in different ways. Men may describe feeling unable to concentrate at work, not wanting to talk about the loss and feeling socially withdrawn. They will sometimes increase their alcohol intake. Women are more likely to cry and to feel very down and unmotivated. They may feel out of control emotionally, at times wanting to tell their story many times and at other times not wanting to be with people. They often feel scared they will not come through this event.

Every pregnancy loss is individual to you and your partner, if you have one. The loss will affect you differently from others, and so their advice may or may not help. Talking is good, so hopefully you will be able to talk with your partner or to another important person and acknowledge the sorrow you feel.

You may want to do something to commemorate the hope this potential child brought to you. Sometimes this may involve planting a shrub, other times it is packaging up all the results of that pregnancy and putting them safely in a top cupboard so they are out of sight but still there. No matter how early the loss, it is a loss and brings with it sadness that you have the right to feel. This loss and sadness will pass with time, and one of the ways to move through it is to get back to your previous activities and life. The structure and routines of our lives can support us in times of troubles.

Age and miscarriage

Increasing age means an increasing likelihood of miscarriage. While women under 35 have a 1 in 5 chance of miscarriage, between 35 and 44 the likelihood of miscarriage is 1 in 3, then by 45 the chance is 1 in 2 or greater. It is rare for a woman at 45 to get pregnant with her own eggs, and the miscarriage rate is high because egg quality declines with increasing age. This is largely because of chromosomal abnormalities.

While men's sperm does deteriorate over 45, the impact this has on miscarriage is not known.

Recurrent miscarriages

A very few women are in the sad situation of having repeated miscarriages (generally regarded as three or more). This can be very traumatic for the women or couples involved. The roller coaster of hope and despair are hard to tolerate and cause emotions that people outside of the situation may find hard to understand.

While some relatively simple tests (genetic/chromosomal/endocrine/hormonal factors) and talking about lifestyle factors can be done to exclude some issues for both the woman and the man, generally there is often no simple answer as to why it is happening. Seeing a specialist and having the tests done may be reassuring for couples.

Couples who have recurrent miscarriages can benefit from fertility counselling to talk about the impact of the repetitive nature of their loss, and to try to identify the things that may help them on this difficult journey. Counselling may help alleviate the anxiety and depression many of these people struggle with.

Later pregnancy loss

This is a unique situation that fortunately happens for only a few people. In most of life, and for most people, death happens after a series of memories have been built up around the deceased person. These memories may provide comfort and allow conversation about the loss.

Later pregnancy loss or stillbirth occurs when the parents are looking forward to building these memories and are hopeful and full of anticipation. Grieving for a baby whose arrival has been looked forward to eagerly and anticipated with joy and now is not experienced is difficult. The loss is not connected to experiences but to dreams and wishes, hopes and fantasies. These may have been shared between the couple, who are likely to be prepared to be parents. Instead they need to find a way to acknowledge the child and to get through the legal requirements (such as registering the child), the autopsy and people's reactions. Both parents will be grieving and may find it difficult to support the other partner and provide for their needs.

There are a number of investigations that are designed to look for a cause of later pregnancy loss or stillbirth. Parents may feel guilt that they have to go through this and wonder if they have contributed to the death. While this investigation is necessary if a future pregnancy is to be attempted, it is not easy for the couple to get through.

Emily and Shane

Emily and Shane lost their much-wanted baby at 26 weeks. Emily went into labour, and while they got to the hospital relatively quickly the doctors were unable to find a heartbeat for the baby. They went to the labour room as birthing the baby was the option given to them.

Their child was born looking small and perfect. Emily and Shane were pleased to be able to hold and love him for a few hours before the staff took him away. Some time later, the staff returned the baby and suggested the couple invite their families to meet him if they wished.

Emily felt they were truly cared for and supported while in the hospital, and the staff took good care to explain to them the process they would need to go through before they got their son home for a funeral or cremation. The couple found it very distressing to think of their child being autopsied.

When their son came home they had chosen to have a small ceremony with family and close friends to farewell him. They had some photos, footprints and handprints taken.

Emily sought counselling several times in the weeks following. She commented she had no one to talk with about her son and all the hopes she had for him and for them as a family. She wept and talked, often repeating things. Sometimes Shane came with her, but he felt as if he had some peace with the loss and her distress made him feel helpless. Gradually she felt able to participate in their life together, firstly in small ways like supermarket shopping and then getting back to work, and some months later taking tentative steps back into a social life.

Emily and Shane took their time to grieve and to find a place for their son in their lives. Then they went on to have two other children.

Grieving

When grief is for the loss of a pregnancy or a child that has not been alive in the world it is complicated and may take some time. The loss is intangible and is often not publicly acknowledged, and there are few rituals for mourning. This results in a perceived lack of support or understanding of the situation. Friends and family may not be able to comfortably speak about the pregnancy or child, and the message the grieving parents feel they receive is that they should just get on with life. This sense of the loss as a topic of conversation to avoid is distressing to the parents.

Each person has an individual way of coping with grief. Women and men grieve differently—this does not mean one grieves more or less for the lost child and opportunities, it is just different. The way we grieve depends on many factors, such as past experience of grief, upbringing and attitudes to grief and emotion and culture.

Things to think about

- How can you acknowledge the loss to yourself?
- In what ways will you remember this hoped-for child?
- Who can you talk with about this loss and feel safe and not judged?
- How can you ensure this loss does not threaten your relationship, and what can you do to support your partner?

- What activities can you undertake that bring back the feeling of being part of the world again?

Things that might be helpful

- Keeping pictures of the scans or photos to help remind you the pregnancy was real.
- Writing a small record of the feelings and dreams that occurred before the miscarriage, including changes in the body, blood test results and any other things that changed.
- Accepting all the memory things the staff offer to set up—foot-and handprints, photos, time with the child. You have one opportunity to get these, and can always choose not to keep them at a later time.
- Considering some level of memorial activity, such as planting a tree or shrub.
- Taking very good care of yourself and beginning activities such as walks and good meals early on, as these will help progress other activities.

Chapter 19

A family affair

Everyone needs family and/or friends at times of stress. The hope is generally that the people we are close to will provide the support and caring that we need in times of struggle. Often the couple are so impacted by their infertility they cannot see the effect on others in their family and friendship groups. If you, as family or friends, have some understanding of infertility and its impact on people, it will help you support them in the best possible way. Be aware you will need to look after yourselves also.

Family and friends do well to avoid making suggestions or broad statements like 'You will be fine, I know you will have children', as they say this without understanding the journey the people involved are about to undertake. Comments such as 'This must be hard for you', 'I am happy to listen and support you', or 'What can I do to help you?' are much more likely to support and help. These comments acknowledge the capacity of the couple or person to run their lives but signal the desire to be alongside them.

Many family and friends want to understand the issues their special person is going through and would like to research the issue. They are advised to stay with New Zealand websites—clinic websites are informative and available to everyone. The consumer group FertilityNZ's website is free to join and has excellent information. These sites are highly appropriate to the issues and treatments offered in New Zealand. I offer a cautionary word about blogs as many of the people on them have an agenda, which means they will have biases that may be unhelpful.

Family need to recognise they will be affected by their family member's situation. They see the losses and the suffering of their young people. Family also feel the loss of their hopes and dreams. They may be hoping to be grandparents or aunties and uncles, and seeing that this may not happen means they have their own grief. It is hard to keep our own grief in check while supporting the people in the centre of this fertility journey. Other family members need to acknowledge to themselves their potential loss and their sadness for the difficulty their loved ones are experiencing. This may make it hard to celebrate another child's arrival within the family when you know how bereft one of your loved ones is about their situation.

Henry and Claire

Henry and Claire were in their early thirties when they decided to have children. They were planning to have three children as they both grew up in families of three and thought that the best number. They stopped using contraception and spent six months happily trying for a pregnancy without success, but also not worrying too much as they knew it might take a while. After six months they began to feel concerned and a bit stressed about the lack of success and the time going by. Probably the biggest issue was that they both had siblings who had announced pregnancies and they were getting comments from family about it being their turn. They had not told their families they were having troubles as they felt this was their problem, but it all came to a head when Claire went to visit their new niece and burst into tears while holding the child.

Once the problem was in the open, their families tried gently to give them suggestions to help and tried to be compassionate about it. Unfortunately each family member raised the issue when they saw them, and Henry and Claire started to avoid being with their families. They felt as if they were only seen as the problem, and recognised their families were struggling but did not know how to help them.

Henry's parents, Marjorie and Stan, with Henry and Claire's consent, came to counselling as they felt they needed to have a safe place to express their sadness and find out how they and their families could best support the couple.

Marjorie and Stan had had three children and Henry was their first. When Henry and Claire struggled to have children the whole family was impacted. Henry's siblings dreaded telling Henry and Claire about pregnancies. They were constantly guarding their words around Henry and Claire and feeling constrained about showing the joy they felt in being pregnant and in their children.

Marjorie and Stan wanted to help the young couple, but it seemed every bit of advice or kindness was wrong. They watched the impact on other family members and felt they all could not really enjoy the pregnancies, babies and grandbabies, especially when with Henry and Claire. Marjorie and Stan did not feel free to talk about their grandchildren any time Henry and Claire were present. Marjorie wept as she talked about their sense of helplessness, of being one step back from the action and not being able to hear first-hand from the doctor what was going on (Marjorie was a nurse) and not being able to question the couple so that she felt informed.

Stan looked after his wife and occasionally joined the discussion. We talked about the situation and acknowledged their feelings and grief. I asked them to reflect on the role they had wanted their parents to take in their relationship when they were young. This helped them realise they needed to support only and not try to drive the situation. We talked about the importance of listening without giving any advice, to provide Henry and Claire with a place to vent their frustration and sadness. We discussed Henry and Claire's need for autonomy. Finally we talked about the whole family and about Marjorie and Stan helping Henry's siblings to understand. They needed to include Henry and Claire in activities and to talk about things other than children and infertility so Henry and Claire felt like valued family members and not a problem.

Henry and Claire had treatment, conceived and had their first child with

> a couple of embryos frozen for a subsequent attempt. They commented during treatment how much it had helped them all to have a plan for the family.

Understanding the impact of infertility

New Zealand is a family-based society, and people grow up believing they will be able to replicate the lifestyle they had in childhood and to share with children the good things they recall from their childhood. When they discover they are going to struggle to become parents some of the founding assumptions about their future are challenged. Their core values, such as the place of a family in their future, are in doubt. They are unsure how they can maintain strong relationships with people who are successful in having families. Not being sure about how to continue to belong to groups whose activities focus around children is a common comment from people grappling with fertility problems.

Most women and many men see parenting as part of their life journey, alongside their career. Some women have jobs that they know will provide good parental leave and part-time work to return to at the end of the parental leave. In some couples it is the man who will be the stay-at-home parent, and who has these expectations challenged.

Surrounding most people who are struggling with a lack of pregnancy are family, friends and workmates who are announcing pregnancies and excitedly wanting to share the pregnancies with others. When people are striving to get pregnant they do not want to be left out when others share about being pregnant. Knowing significant information about other family and friends is part of being included in that group.

There is a boundary for infertile couples, and they need family and friends to be sensitive about including them but not giving a lot of detail. Being part of lengthy discussions about pregnancy, and often complaints about how hard it is or how unwell the woman is feeling, is particularly hard for an infertile woman to bear. Remembering that life is about more than pregnancy and children and ensuring you share moments about other aspects in life is a kindness when talking with those struggling to conceive.

Sometimes in an effort to help, friends or family may point out that having children is not always fun and a good time. Pregnancy can be difficult, birth tricky and children may test parents as they grow. Talking about this is unhelpful for those who desperately wish to have children and see the joy they bring other people.

Our society has a number of celebrations based around families—Christmas, Easter, Guy Fawkes are some. These celebrations can be particularly hard on those struggling with infertility, as they centre around children and therefore emphasise childlessness, often causing another level of sadness and grief. Mother's and Father's Days are particularly difficult for those struggling with infertility as acknowledging their own parents brings into focus their childless state. Sometimes family need to understand that their people who are struggling to have children may wish to only take part in some of the celebration, or perhaps miss a year.

There are commonly held beliefs and myths around infertility, and these are mentioned in 'Chapter 4: Beliefs and values—how these can help or hinder'. It is useful for families to recognise that sometimes their understanding may not be supported by the science and is not useful to the couple.

Things to think about for family and friends

- It is helpful to have some information, but it is not helpful for you to give advice or to put the couple under pressure to change behaviours.
- Be available to be a listening ear, but ensure you let them own the problem.
- Encourage them to seek professional help early. The standard recommended time of seeking help

when there is no conception after 6–12 months is important. If you are young (in your twenties) you are more likely to conceive easily, so getting to the clinic early is worthwhile to exclude problems. If you are over 35 you need to get the investigations going as these things can take time and your fertility window is getting smaller, especially if you want more than one child. Government funding is not available when a woman is over 40, so getting to the specialist earlier gives you a chance to access this.

- Families can offer support by changing their lifestyles to help couples make changes. Take a look at your lifestyle and see if there are things you can do to help—men and women can stop smoking, vaping and using recreational drugs as they all affect both sperm and egg production. Be moderate about caffeine and alcohol intake.
- Go to New Zealand websites to get a bit informed. This will help you understand the couple's

investigations and treatment, but make sure you allow them to be the experts in their treatment and lives. FertilityNZ has wonderful information for free on its website.

Things that might be helpful

- Listen—just let people talk. Maybe the couple have said it all before, but being prepared to listen again tells them you are trying to understand and you care.
- Do not offer suggestions or advice—ask them what you can do to help. Generally they will just want you to be there.
- There is a high emotional toll to being unable to have a child, then having treatment. Don't be scared of tears. A hug and some tissues help.
- Life before children and infertility involved doing and talking about other things. Encourage them to do some of these things again, and limit the time you spend talking about your pregnancy or children.

- Invite them to special occasions such as birthdays—they are quite capable of deciding whether to attend or if they can't manage it. Don't put pressure on to attend.
- Adoption is infrequent these days for various reasons. Be wary of suggesting or encouraging it as it is unlikely to happen.
- Take care of yourself—supporting others has a cost and it is important to be around for what may be a long journey.

Chapter 20

Living without children

I acknowledge that almost all the people I counselled at the clinic wanted to parent as their first choice. There were a small number of couples or individuals over the two decades of my counselling who wanted to talk about life without children as a first option. I also have friends and family who have chosen for whatever reason to not be parents.

There have been couples who have come to talk about their desire to not parent and the enormous pressure they feel to please their families. These people wish to get on with their lives without severing their bond with their important people. This is a conflict that they often have no safe place to work through.

Sometimes people seek counselling because they have no picture of children in their lives, or they don't especially like children. These people are often reconciled to not parenting, and just wish for ways to have the world understand this is a choice and they do not want pressure around this choice. In fact they often would prefer not to discuss it, and just to be accepted.

The decision to accept not being a parent is a big one. In countries such as New Zealand and Australia society and its religious backdrop is based around children. The lives of most people are family-based—they are involved with their grandparents, parents, sisters and brothers and often nieces and nephews. This involves celebrations such as birthdays and Christmases in which they may wish to participate. Often these celebrations, and especially Christmas and Easter, are focused around the youngest generation of the family. To those who wanted to parent, this may be a painful reminder that they do not have children to be loved and spoilt, firstly by them and then by the rest of the family.

Often people have survived the baby showers and births and naming ceremonies of their family's children using the fantasy that one day it will be their turn. These hopes and dreams are also lost and sad to give up. It is difficult to find a replacement dream. Often the people who cannot or do not want to have children also have to help their important others accept this.

With so much of life accommodating children of all ages and the sharing of their accomplishments or trials, it is hard for childless couples to find people and a place that acknowledges their situation.

When people have tried hard to parent, they may have spent a lot of time, emotion and money in the effort. As they reach the end of their treatment, whether there is nothing further available in treatment or they simply feel they have reached the end of their emotional and financial resources, they feel sadness and a sense of being cheated by life. For so long they have had the roller coaster of hope and disappointment and generally they are weary of the struggle by the time they get to recognising they cannot continue. Their task at this point is to work towards what else will make their lives worthwhile and to begin to plan the move forward.

Accepting that they will not be parents requires rethinking the daily expectations and taking the focus off the routine that fertility treatment has imposed. It involves stopping reading the blogs and websites about becoming pregnant. Taking out of the phone any reminders or dates that focus on fertility. This may leave a gap in especially the woman's life, as she may have been charting her periods and fertile times diligently for some years. By stopping these activities she is acknowledging the change in her life. The difficult part is to find something to fill the gap that feels worthwhile. To fill this gap the person needs to consider the things they enjoyed doing before trying to having children became the focus. Whatever the first activities are to fill this gap, they are often a short-term measure, and there will be other things to try.

Michelle and Anthony

Michelle and Anthony had had a long and stable relationship since their early working days. They decided to start a family around five years before they sought help, having always acknowledged they wanted to parent. Initially they were unconcerned about their lack of success, however they started reading about fertility and realised they needed to get help before age was an issue. The fertility specialist found Michelle had endometriosis despite her lack of symptoms, and recommended they have IVF to try to get around this. The specialist also told them of Anthony's low sperm count—not only did he not have as many sperm as desirable, they did not swim well and had some odd shapes. This would mean that as well as IVF they would need some testing done on the sperm, and then ICSI.

They had a number of unsuccessful treatments before donor treatment was suggested. This felt like a step too far for them, and they decided to talk about creating a life without children. When they talked with family they received opposition and were told they would regret the decision later in life. It was at this point they came to the counsellor, mostly because they could not think of anyone else they could talk with.

In counselling Michelle raised that their first choice was to have children together, but when it involved so many professionals and the drugs she disliked taking, she started to think about options. Anthony was glad to hear of her talking about being child-free. He had taken time to think about this and he knew they had family who would disagree with the decision. As a couple they needed strategies to move forward.

The very simple decision-making tool of looking at the pros and cons of children and being child-free served this couple well. They then decided they needed to find satisfying activities. They looked at their lives pre-fertility treatment and got some ideas from there of things they thought they might like to try again.

Anthony decided to consider some extra training or a career change, and Michelle supported him in this.

Gradually they made new friends who did not have children, and their families accepted their decision, and the couple were able to enjoy their nieces and nephews as they grew older.

Finding alternative values and lifestyles, including friends who will understand and who appreciate similar activities, is challenging. Discovering what will be fulfilling for each person is sometimes a mission. Then there is feeling comfortable explaining this to those friends and family who are important.

There is no magic formula in deciding, when someone has wished to have children, that they need to accept it is not going to happen. There are however some very handy hints that will help people get through the initial hard stage.

People who go to a counsellor to talk about closure often have reached their 'line in the sand'. This imaginary line says anything more is a step too far. There are many reasons why this may occur. Emotionally, people get exhausted by fertility treatment. They find having life on hold frustrating and unsatisfying. They dislike the hope-and-disappointment cycle they have been in. Other times people have reached the end of their financial resources and cannot fund any more treatment. Or it may be that the couple or even one person may not be able to cope with the thought of further treatment and the control this has on their lives. Sometimes it is the clinic that says they are unable to help any further. Other times the next level of treatment crosses the couple or the person's boundaries and is against their beliefs and value system.

Grief is the most commonly felt emotion as the person or couple realises they are leaving treatment and not going back to the clinic. The grief can be a composite of many emotions—sorrow, guilt, frustration, anger, despair, depression, regret, loneliness, resentment, isolation and helplessness. It can be a strong feeling or just a niggle. Grief can be simple or very complex. It can come in waves or be constant. There is no 'normal' for grief—we each do it in our own way and according to the loss we are feeling. There is no right or wrong.

There may also sometimes be a sense of relief of having this phase over and being able to move forward. There is often fatigue—fertility fatigue—and the tiredness takes a while to dissipate.

Acknowledging that we feel these emotions is a useful start. Once a person recognises they are sad they can then validate the emotion by saying—internally if necessary—'I am sad because I would have liked to have children and realise it is unlikely to happen' or 'I feel alone and lonely because all my friends have children and talk about them all the time and I can't join in'.

There are a number of things that seem to help many people as they are grieving the loss of being a parent. Things such as having a pet to love, or exercise, which keeps the body moving and also helps the emotions move along so we do not get stuck on a thought or emotion. Recognising we all have a repertoire of activities that we have enjoyed in the past, and trying these out again to see if they are still interesting and helpful now. These activities may be creative and cognitive or practical and concrete, so at the end you have a product to enjoy—activities like building a raised garden, making a cake, stitching, fixing something around home. The satisfaction from seeing a job on the way or done is strong. It gives us control over a part of our lives when our fertility has been out of control.

Trying a new activity is very energising and can help us get through the hard times. The challenge of having success at this activity compensates somewhat for the lack of success in the fertility area.

As time goes by we grow used to the childless state. We do not forget we would have liked to parent, but we find lives that provide us with other satisfactions. Sometimes we find ways of loving children we had not expected to find, such as being the best aunty or uncle or godparent to a child who needs us. Other times we find other ways to contribute to society.

My favourite comment and one I have used a lot in my life comes from Virginia Satir, a family therapist. I have paraphrased it here: 'Life is not what we want it to be, it is what it is. It is what we do with it that matters.'

Things to think about

* Do you just need to take a break from treatment or do you need to stop?
* Identify the reasons you have reached this point, to help understand why this time has arrived.
* Who are the people in your life who accept your decisions?
* Do you have any friends without children, who you could spend more time with?
* Jobs take up a big portion of every day. Do not make change too quickly, but consider whether your job is giving you satisfaction and achievement.

- What activities can you be successful with to balance the lack of success of fertility treatment?

Things that might be helpful

- Finding someone to talk with if you do not have a partner—someone who will listen but not give advice.
- Developing some statements to fend off others' advice and opinions, such as 'I do not want to talk about this right now' or 'This is my/our decision and I/we would like you to accept it'.
- Making a list of activities you would like to try or know you have enjoyed in the past but stopped doing.
- Exercising—it helps move emotions onwards.
- Giving yourself permission to read a book or watch a movie to distract yourself.

Appendix

The laws influencing fertility treatment

As with all medical services there are a number of Acts of Parliament that influence all aspects of treatment. New Zealand has signed a number of international human rights covenants, conventions and protocols. This ensures it has international obligations to uphold the rights of its people.

Te Tiriti o Waitangi, the Treaty of Waitangi

Te Tiriti o Waitangi, the Treaty of Waitangi, was first signed on 6 February 1840, and is the foundation document for New Zealand society. It frames the political relationships between Māori and Pākehā, recognising that Māori rights must be considered in other legal frameworks. The fertility legal documents all recognise and adhere to the Treaty of Waitangi. Fertility clinics, while operating under Western medical practices, try to be inclusive in the practical aspects that will ensure Māori and other nationalities can feel comfortable accepting treatment within the clinic.

The Human Rights Act 1993

Our over-riding law affecting every aspect of New Zealand life is the Human Rights Act of 1993, which protects people in New Zealand from discrimination. Unlawful discrimination is when treatment is less favourable than others might receive based on age, colour, disability, employment status, ethical belief, ethnic or national origin, family status, marital status, political opinion, race, religious belief, sex or sexual orientation. Fertility clinics ensure they do their best to be as non-discriminatory as possible.

The Human Rights Act is the umbrella Act that all other Acts recognise. When there is a legal need or complaint in the fertility field, the Human Rights Act and the Human Assisted Reproductive Technology Act (see below) interact to look for the wellbeing of all those involved, including the unborn children.

Human Assisted Reproductive Technology Act (HART Act)

Fertility treatment has its own Act, the Human Assisted Reproductive Technology (HART) Act 2004, which takes into account Te Tiriti o Waitangi and The Human Rights Act and sets out the principles to follow for fertility treatment.

The HART Act, along with the Human Rights Act and Te Tiriti o Waitangi, guides the clinics and provides the clinics and their staff with the principles that give fairness and equality while working within the constraints of the Ministry of Health regulations and funding. These principles not only care for the patients using the clinic, they ensure that staff work within boundaries which keep the patients, staff and clinics safe.

The HART Act recognises some procedures are 'established', and clinics can proceed with these treatments automatically (e.g. IVF and most donations of gametes). Clinics provide the Ministry of Health with data about these procedures. It is assumed the clinics will care for the safety and wellbeing of all people, including the unborn child(ren) involved in the treatments.

Section 32 of the HART Act requires two advisory committees to guide the clinics. The first, the Advisory Committee on Assisted Reproductive Technology, ACART, issues guidelines and advice to ECART, the Ethics Committee on Assisted Reproductive Technology. ECART uses the guidelines for the case-by-case consideration of applications for treatment that is not an 'established' treatment. These treatments, such as embryo donation and surrogacy, may affect more than one person, couple or family and existing children, and are vetted because their consequences are lifelong for all participants, including existing and hoped-for children. The ethical approval is designed to ensure all parties have considered the implications of the treatments and, in cases such as surrogacy, have a robust enough relationship to be able to problem-solve should it be needed. The principle of doing no harm is important in these considerations.

Within the HART Act, section 3 contains directions for the clinics to collect certain specified non-identifying information from the donor, and this will be available to those using the gametes, to the children who result from the use and to their guardians. It requires that the clinics notify the Department of Births, Deaths and Marriages (BDM) about the birth of a child so the Donor Register can hold the genetic parentage information about each child born through donor insemination. The identity of the donor is available as of right to the young person at 18 years. The Donor Register is a closed register holding the information for the young person, unless there are exceptional circumstances. The principle of the right of a young person to their genetic information is stated within the HART Act.

The purposes of the HART Act are:

(a)   to secure the benefits of assisted reproductive procedures, established procedures, and human reproductive research for individuals and for society in general by taking appropriate measures for the protection and promotion of the health, safety, dignity, and rights of all individuals, but particularly those of women and children, in the use of these procedures and research:

(b)   to prohibit unacceptable reproductive procedures and unacceptable human reproductive research:

(c)   to prohibit certain commercial transactions relating to human reproduction:

(d)   to provide a robust and flexible framework for regulating and guiding the performance of assisted reproductive procedures and the conduct of human reproductive research:

(e)   to prohibit the performance of assisted reproductive procedures (other than established procedures) or the conduct of human reproductive research without the continuing approval of the ethics committee:

(f)   to establish a comprehensive information-keeping regime to ensure that people born from donated embryos or donated cells can find out about their genetic origins.

The principles of the Act are:

(a)   the health and well-being of children born as a result of the performance of an assisted reproductive procedure or an established procedure should be an important consideration in all decisions about that procedure:

(b)   the human health, safety, and dignity of present and future generations should be preserved and promoted:

(c)   while all persons are affected by assisted human reproductive procedures and established procedures, women, more than men, are directly and significantly affected by their application, and the health and well-being of women must be protected in the use of these procedures:

(d) no assisted human reproductive procedure should be performed on an individual and no human reproductive research should be conducted on an individual unless the individual has made an informed choice and given informed consent:

(e) donor offspring should be made aware of their genetic origins and be able to access information about those origins:

(f) the needs, values, and beliefs of Māori should be considered and treated with respect:

(g) the different ethical, spiritual, and cultural perspectives in society should be considered and treated with respect.

Gamete and embryo storage

Fertility clinics are able to store eggs, sperm and embryos for 10 years from the time of their creation if the embryos are made from the gametes of the people using them. If there is a donor involved in making a stored embryo, the 10 years begins when the donor donates the gametes.

People are able to apply to extend their storage period by putting in an application to ECART for an extension to the storage, before the previous storage expires.

Ethical approval

There are a series of situations where ethical approval is required before treatment can take place. Currently these include surrogacy, donation of embryos, use of donated eggs with donated sperm, donation of gametes between certain family members, extension to the storage of gametes and embryos, and research projects.

In New Zealand these treatments have to have case-by-case ethical approval from ECART. The guidelines for these treatments are readily available for anyone to peruse, and the applications are completed by clinic staff and lawyers as advocates of patients as part of the non-identifying application to ECART.

ECART consists of members who represent a broad range of disciplines, professions and interests, including expertise in fertility medicine, bioethics, health and disability, Māori health and consumer advocacy. The committee meets about six times a year to consider applications. They receive them a month prior to the meeting, and they release their decision around a month after the meeting. It is not until the clinics receive approval from ECART that they can proceed with treatment.

Forbidden Acts

The HART Act informs about which procedures and treatments cannot be undertaken. This includes some research and sex selection of embryos, and it places boundaries around advertising and payment within treatment.

Other considerations

There are other laws which influence fertility considerations, such as the Care of Children Act 2004, which has as its primary purpose to promote children's welfare and best interests and facilitate their development.

The Adoption Act 1955, and its subsequent amendments, are important in applications for surrogacy. Intending parents currently have to adopt the child from the birth parents (surrogates) despite the child being usually but not always genetically from at least one of the intending parents. At the time of writing there is a Member's Bill in front of Parliament hoping to change this law. This has not currently yet been considered by Parliament.

Glossary and acronyms

ACART—Advisory Committee on Assisted Reproductive Technology—provides advice to the Minister of Health and issues guidelines and provides advice to ECART on procedures and research

AMH— anti-mullerian hormone—hormone test to check ovarian reserve

BMI—body mass index—a person's weight in kilograms divided by the square of height in metres

biochemical pregnancy—early pregnancy detected by biochemical pregnancy test; term generally used when pregnancy does not continue

blastocyst—an embryo five to seven days after fertilisation, which consists of an outer mass of cells that may form the placenta and an inner mass that may form the foetus

DNA—deoxyribonucleic acid—the carrier of genetic information, it carries fundamental and distinctive characteristics of someone or something

D&C—dilation and curettage—a small procedure done under anaesthetic to remove the tissues of pregnancy

donor embryo—unused IVF embryos after completion of a family that are gifted to another person or couple

donor oocyte—when a woman undergoes IVF to gift her eggs to another woman

donor sperm—sperm given by a man (donor) for use by a woman who is not his partner; may be used in IUI or IVF

Downs syndrome—a genetic disorder in chromosome 21 that causes developmental and intellectual delays

ECART—Ethics Committee on Assisted Reproductive Technology—a committee using the guidelines of ACART that provides case-by-case approval for some treatments that are not 'established' practices (e.g. surrogacy)

EDCs—endocrine disrupting chemicals—substances found in natural and manufactured materials; they can interfere with the body's normal functioning

endometriosis—the presence of endometrial tissue outside of the uterus

foetus—an embryo from eight weeks until birth

FSH—follicle-stimulating hormone—a hormone produced by the pituitary gland that stimulates the ripening of an ovum or egg

gametes—eggs or sperm

GP—general practitioner or family doctor

HART Act—Human Assisted Reproductive Technology Act—the 2004 law that secures the benefits of assisted reproductive technologies and prohibits unacceptable practices

hCG—human chorionic gonadotropin—the hormone used to measure pregnancy

ICSI—intracytoplasmic sperm injection—the injection of a single sperm into an egg

I U I — i n t r a u t e r i n e insemination—when sperm is placed into a woman's uterus

I V F — i n vitro fertilisation—fertilisation of eggs by sperm outside of the body; the process involves the stimulation of the ovaries to produce a number of eggs, collection of the eggs, fertilisation of the eggs, the growing of any potential embryos in the laboratory and replacement and/or freezing of embryos

Klinefelter syndrome—a random genetic anomaly that means a man has an extra X chromosome and probably low testosterone and no sperm

mindfulness—a way of paying attention to what is presently occurring; when we are being mindful we lower stress and feel less anxious and depressed

miscarriage—or spontaneous abortion, is the loss of a foetus before 20 weeks. Typically it happens in the first trimester (or first three months) of pregnancy

ovulation induction—a treatment to induce ovulation when it does not occur naturally

PGD—preimplantation genetic diagnosis—the testing of blastocyst embryos for genetic conditions

PGS—preimplantation genetic screening—testing of embryos to check they have the correct number of chromosomes

pituitary gland—a small gland attached to the base of the brain that controls the activity of most other hormone-secreting glands

polycystic ovaries—enlarged ovaries with small cysts around the outer edges

SCSA—sperm chromatin structure assay—a test to check levels of DNA damage of sperm while in the testes

semen analysis—the study of semen under a powerful microscope to look at sperm numbers and morphology (shape, size, swimming capacity)

surgical sperm retrieval—a fine-needle aspiration to remove sperm directly from the testes

Bibliography

ACART Guidelines for Family Gamete Donation, Embryo Donation, the Use of Donated Eggs with Donated Sperm and Clinic Assisted Surrogacy, ACART, Wellington, September 2020.

ACART Supplementary Information to the Donation and Surrogacy Guideline (draft), ACART, Wellington, August 2020.

American College of Obstetricians and Gynaecologists FAQs, 'Having a Baby After 35: How aging affects fertility and pregnancy', https://www.acog.org/Patients/FAQs/Having-a-Baby-After-Age-35-How-Aging-Affects-Fertility-and-Pregnancy?, accessed October 2020.

Adrienne, Helen, 'Shattered Self-esteem: A byproduct of infertility', https://www.huffpost.com/entry/shattered-self-esteem-a-by_b_11458492, Huffpost.com, accessed 6 December 2019.

Bannan, Christine, and Winnie Duggan, *Be Fertile with Your Infertility: Creative ways to acknowledge the infertility journey using ceremony and ritual,* Bateson Publishing, Wellington, 2008.

Birdsall, Dr Mary, ed., *Making Babies: The New Zealand guide to getting pregnant,* David Bateman, Auckland, 2009.

Blagdon, Jenny, Annette Dixon and Robyn Scott, *The Elusive Dream: New Zealanders' stories of living with infertility,* J Blagdon, Wellington, 2002.

Covington, Sharon N. and Linda Hammer Burns, *Infertility Counselling: A comprehensive handbook for clinicians,* 2nd ed., Cambridge University Press, New York, 2009.

Day, Jody, *Living the Life Unexpected,* Bluebird Books for Life, London, 2016.

Deveraux, Lara L. and Ann Jackoway Hammerman, *Infertility and Identity: New strategies for treatment,*

Jossey-Bass Publishers, San Francisco, 1998.

Eck Menning, Barbara, *Infertility: A guide for the childless couple*, Prentice-Hall, New Jersey, 1977.

Extend Fertility, 'Fertility on Hold: What you can do while you wait', https://ex tendfertility.com/what-you-can-do-now-trying-to-conceive-later/, Extendfertility .com, accessed 24 April 2020.

Fertility Associates, *Pathway to a Child*, March 2020.

Fertility Society of Australia, 'How to Avoid Chemicals That Can Reduce Fertility', https://www.yourfertility.org. au/sites/default/files/2018-08/How_to_ avoid_chemicals_that_can_reduce_fertil ity.pdf, Australian Government and Victorian Government Department of Health and Human Services, accessed October 2020.

Frank, Michael, 'What Almost Four Years in the Land of Infertility Taught Me About Waiting', Time.com, https://time

.com/5732068/infertility-waiting/, accessed 18 November 2019.

Kidspot, 'The Impact of Age on Fertility', https://kidspot.co.nz/pregnancy/age-and-fertility/, Kidspot.com, accessed August 2020.

Mental Health Foundation, 'Finding Balance: Te whare tapa whā', https://www.mentalhealth.org.nz/assets/Working-Well/WS-finding-balance-individual.pdf, accessed 2019.

Mental Health Foundation, 'Five Ways to Wellbeing', https://www.mentalhealth.org.nz/home/ways-to-wellbeing/, accessed June 2020.

Neimeyer, Robert A., Darcy L. Harris, Howard R. Winokuer and Gordon F. Thornton, *Grief and Bereavement in Contemporary Society,* Routledge Publishers, New York, 2011.

New Zealand Institute of Wellbeing and Resilience, Dr Lucy Hone and Dr Denise Quinlan, 'Real-time Resilience Strategies for Coping with Coronavirus', https://n

ziwr.co.nz/wp-content/uploads/2020/03/NZIWR_Real-time_Resilience_Coping_with_Coronavirus.pdf, accessed September 2020.

New Zealand Law Commission, *New Issues in Legal Parenthood,* Law Commission Report 88, New Zealand Law Commission, Wellington, 2005.

Rupnow, Jana LPC, *Three Makes Baby: How to parent your donor conceived child,* Rupnow and Associates, Dallas, 27 August 2018.

Saunders, Sue, *Infertility: A guide for New Zealanders,* Penguin, Auckland, 1998.

Shapiro, Dani, *Inheritance: A memoir of genealogy, paternity and love,* Daunt Books, New York, 2019.

www.ingramcontent.com/pod-product-compliance
Lightning Source LLC
Chambersburg PA
CBHW011225210326
41598CB00040B/7319